HAND and FOOT REFLEXOLOGY

A Self-Help Guide

by Kevin and Barbara Kunz

Edited by Kenneth L. Shoemaker

PRENTICE HALL PRESS

New York London Toronto Sydney Tokyo

Copyright © 1984 by Kevin and Barbara Kunz
All rights reserved, including the right of reproduction
in whole or in part in any form.

Published in 1987 by Prentice Hall Press
A Division of Simon & Schuster, Inc.
Gulf + Western Building
One Gulf + Western Plaza
New York, NY 10023

Originally published by Prentice-Hall, Inc.
Illustrations by Barbara Kunz
Typesetting, Paste-up and Design by Betty Colvin
Design Consultant: Peter Kunz

PRENTICE HALL PRESS is a trademark of Simon & Schuster, Inc.

Library of Congress Cataloging-in-Publication Data

Kunz, Kevin.
   Hand and foot reflexology

   Bibliography: p.
   Includes index.
   1. Reflexotherapy.   I. Kunz, Barbara.   II. Shoe-
maker, Kenneth L.   III. Title.
RM723.R43K864   1984   615.8'22   84-11720
ISBN 0-13-383589-8
ISBN 0-13-383571-5 (pbk.)

Manufactured in the United States of America

10   9   8   7   6

Books by Kevin and Barbara Kunz
THE COMPLETE GUIDE TO FOOT REFLEXOLOGY (1982)
HAND AND FOOT REFLEXOLOGY: A Self-Help Guide (1984)
HAND REFLEXOLOGY WORKBOOK: How To Work on
   Someone's Hands (1985)
THE PRACTITIONER'S GUIDE TO REFLEXOLOGY (1985)

TABLE OF CONTENTS

PREFACE

To date, traditional reflexology has left open the question: why does reflexology work? The effects generally listed up to now have been: improved circulation; normalized gland and organ function; and, inducing a state of relaxation. However, there has been no well defined or defensible answer as to why working on the feet and hands yield such remarkable results.

Such a vague and unclear posture has prompted us to search for answers. A former student and a good friend, Ruth Hahn, pointed us in the direction of sensory experience as the basis for our research. She is the director of the Miami County Rehabilitation Center for Brain-Injured Adults and Children in Piqua, Ohio. She had applied reflexology as a major component in an overall program of sensory stimulation. Our conversations with her about problems we encountered in one client's case began our education in the sensory system and its function. We soon decided to become "interested self-researchers" as Ruth had done. Our attention was then turned to scientific literature. The feet seemed to have such a fundamental relationship with the rest of the body that there was likely to be at least some reference in research papers or other works.

In actuality, the first encounter occurred in a standard human anatomy book. That is where the word "proprioception" popped up. As we read on, we knew a connection had been found. Proprioceptive definitions mentioned the bottom of the feet repeatedly, indicating that the feet apparently provide very important information in the body's communication system and routinely exchange information with the rest of the body.

Besides this fundamental relationship between foot and body, further searching revealed the foot's contribution to the body's overall state of readiness. In order to accomplish movement efficiently, an overall background of muscular tension, called "tone", must be maintained. The level of tension is pre-set so that one can set different parts of the body to exact positions and these parts can remain in the same position, despite outside forces. "An example of this would be paddling a boat, during which a person sets the degree of force throughout the entire movement." P. 461, *Basic Human Physiology*. Even ordinary walking requires an overall background of tension that is pre-set to accomplish fluid movement.

Tone also determines basic survival. A challenge from outside the body causes an overall increase in the body's tension level. Fight or flight is recognized as a reflexive action that occurs when the body is challenged to extremes. The level of tone in the body is the medium through which this action is accomplished. Tone also serves as a link between the feet, the hands and the internal organs. When the body arouses from sleep to wakefulness or from a resting state to full activity, it is tone which determines how efficiently and quickly this occurs.

Reflexology has always maintained a link between the feet, hands and internal organs. A type of "loop" is commonly described in much of the literature we encountered during our research. Sensory stimulation not only activates and adjusts a response from the muscles and nerves but it also "loops" through the internal organs. Of importance is the proprioceptive messages that cause a "high degree of arousal activity". The automatic activities adjust, along with adjustments throughout the body, to increased demands. In other words, proprioceptive messages from the feet and hands give the body feedback of ongoing external events. The sensory system in turn adjusts in its entirety and then seeks additional information to complete the picture. The internal organs are regulated with adequate levels of fuel to meet the changing demands of the situation.

Survival is the primary function of the body's sensory system. Detecting danger and making an adequate response is the duty of the entire body. Fight or flight (the body's defensive reaction to danger) is a method for increasing the body's readiness in order to make an appropriate response to the situation. Locomotion is a means of making fight or flight possible. It describes the ability to move from place to place, helping to ensure survival.

The stride itself gives evidence that there is a special relationship between the feet and the rest of the body. The foot acts within the sensory system as a sensory organ helping to check changes in the terrain underfoot as they occur. The foot contributes its information to maintain balance under changing conditions. A footstep is a change in the body's attitude and contributes to the overall balance of the body.

As a sensory organ the foot has the ability to adapt to a variety of terrain and conditions. Indeed, shoes and flat surfaces remove the element of challenge to the foot's sensory function. Like any other sensory organ, it tends to lose its adaptability if it is not used.

The foot is also an energy consumer. This consumption is dependent upon its ability to fully utilize its sensory function. Stimulation challenges the foot and re-awakens its abilities to contribute in an efficient operating mode. Practice, for example, makes an athlete's movements more fluid and less energy consuming. Practice makes the foot's function more viable and less energy consuming. Each foot step has the potential for saving energy in the body's finite resources.

Refining tone or the body's readiness is a way of refining movement. The body's tone can be "stuck", like a thermostat, on too high a setting which may mean a reaction of fight and flight to a situation which does not warrant such a reaction. Deliberately using applied pressure on the hands and feet is a way of discovering those pre-set tension levels (tone) and ultimately, of altering them.

Every sensory signal alters tone somewhat. Reflexology is designed to consistently interrupt that tone on a frequent basis. Each interruption leads to a re-evaluation of the situation and a gradual return to a state of balance.

One question left unexplained by reflexology theory is the notion that the image of the body is projected on and represented by the feet. This is the *reiteration theory* (correlating various parts of the feet to various parts of the body). There is precedent for an organizational representation or parliamentation arrangement in the sensory system. In the brain, sensory information is translated into appropriate motor (muscle) responses. This occurs in the sensory-motor cortex. The image projected is a spatial arrangement of body parts reflecting the body image.

Dr. Ralph Alan Dale, in a series of articles relating reflexology to acupuncture, refers to this phenomenon as "reiterative". Reflexology and other systems which project the body whole on a body part (feet, hands, head, face, etc.) are, in fact, based on reiterative theory.

In the very earliest stages of development, the embryo "wires in" the very important sensory organs. This pre-natal "wiring" may be the basis of reiteration. Neurology recognizes each and every cell as being a participant in the body's communication system. A highly developed sensory system capable of the juggling act of human walking would well have evolved a mechanism such as reiteration. More research may clarify the exact nature of reiteration and hopefully identify other participants in the process.

*To Jimmy Romero, Kris Hain, Anne Thomas
and Ruth Hahn.*

*Our thanks to Jan and Rol Schneider,
Sue and Paul Hain, Celena Lueras, Ed Case,
Larry Clemmons, Bob Dallamore, Dave Sayer,
Jill Schneider, JoAnn and Mark Mellone,
Rita Zulka and our parents, Ruth and Kaiser Kunz
and Margaret and Joseph Kurcaba.*

*Our special thanks to Betty Colvin,
Ken Shoemaker, Peter Kunz and Betsy Torjussen
for their fine efforts in the production
of this work.*

INTRODUCTION

After finishing our first book, *The Complete Guide to Foot Reflexology*, our next challenge was to find an answer to the question of how reflexology actually works. Research led us to answers which not only seemed plausible but also spawned the techniques found in this book.

The answer to the question is that any form of sensory signal alters the tone or tension level in the body. Sir Charles Sherrington, the founding father of neurophysiology, is quoted as saying, "A conversation at a cocktail party alters one's life." His observation was made in recognition of the influence of any sensory experience, whether heard, seen or felt.

Traditional reflexology has been practiced as a form of deep-pressure sensory experience applied to the bottoms of the feet. The information provided by such experience is actually vital to the body's ability to walk. While standing or walking, deep pressure to the bottoms of the feet helps the body maintain its position. An enormous amount of information is necessary for the body to maintain an upright, standing position. What makes the task so difficult is having to keep upright on two small pedestals, the feet. The entire body participates and acts in unison in response to deep pressure information from the bottoms of the feet. The demands of this righting principle have given us a link between the feet and the body and served as a source for the incredible responses we have seen to reflexology.

We have used this information not only to help us develop our understanding of the link between the body and the feet, but also to find new ways of interacting with the feet. We came to realize that deep pressure was but one of several locomotive sensory signals which could be replicated and serve as a means of communication with the body. Both the stretch of muscles and the angulation of joints were also sensory signals which provided further exploration for us. As a group, these sensory signals are actually described by the term 'proprioception', the self-perceiving mechanism of the sensory system. All movement requires such perception. Survival itself, the very ability to take flight or fight, is inextricably linked to such a system.

Furthermore, the body's ability to perceive itself is a determinant in its ability to cope with the stresses of daily life. A more accurate body perception results in a finely tuned response to the interactions of the day. Now, we are convinced that interaction with the self perceiving mechanism is possible and can be used to interrupt patterns of stress. Such possibility is intriguing. The potential for the individual lies in the opportunity to interact with the mechanism that regulates stress in the body; in essence, to work with the elements of health, wellness, creativity, fitness, and the quality of life itself.

This book is a manual of possibilities. It is an exploration of sensory experience as applied on a consistent, patterned basis. The many potentials of this approach will be realized through individual application. It is our hope that the user of this information will find his or her exploration to be a rewarding one. □

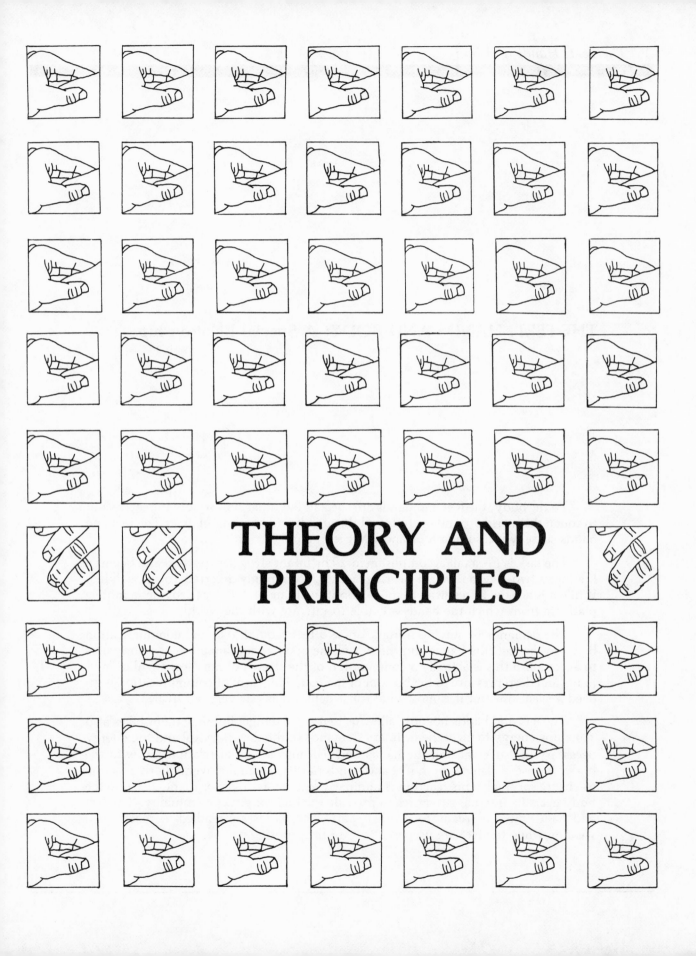

THEORY AND PRINCIPLES

THE FEET, HANDS AND BODY: A Special Relationship

To the body, the feet and hands are special. No other sensory organ reaches out to touch the world around us, to travel through it and to manipulate it. The feet and hands sense what is underfoot and what is in hand.

The task is no small accomplishment. The infant struggles to stand and begins a life-long, two-legged, weight-bearing activity commonly referred to as walking. While it is not the fastest way to move about, walking on two legs provides a mobile platform from which the hands are able to interact with the world.

The demands of staying upright on two feet require a special communication between the feet, the hands and the rest of the body. The "language" the body uses to accomplish this is actually a combination of the stretch of muscles, angulation of joints and deep pressure to the bottom of the feet. This form of communication is indeed a silent one but it is most vital for it determines our very survival.

The feet and hands not only allow us to react to danger but they themselves also consume energy to meet the ordinary demands of the day. Survival and the energy necessary for survival link the hands and feet into a special relationship with the body. In case of danger, both feet and hands participate in the overall body reaction to ensure survival. This reaction is familiarly known as "fight or flight" because the body gears its internal structures to provide the fuel for either eventuality. The feet and hands must be ready to do their part. The hands are readied to reach for a weapon while the feet are prepared to find firm footing or flee.

The inextricable link between hand, foot and body is thus forged. The hands and feet provide the necessary moves while the internal organs provide the fuel. A special communication and relationship is required for such a system.

The system is also a participant in more mundane daily activities. For example, upon waking, the body not only assesses internal organ measurements but it also requests body position information. The feet are polled in this positioning process. The rest of the day is spent in silent dialogue between internal organs and the organs of movement. Every move made, whether to walk, sit, stand, jump, run or skip, requires up-dated information and continual communication. Every move made requires an allocation of the body's energy.

Thus the feet and hands are a part of day-to-day energy consuming activities. This demand forms the basis of very strong links within the body's communication system. To ensure continuity from day to day, the body learns a communication operating pattern. In locomotion, continuity is all important; any interruption in the communication or energy systems could be catastrophic, resulting in, for example, a fall. Therefore the signals of locomotion have major impact on the energy system, the sensory system and the overall tension level of the body. Tension is a state of readiness occurring throughout the body. A footstep requires a great deal of tension to be successful.

This high degree of muscular readiness not only consumes a great deal of energy but it also must be matched by the readiness of the internal environment. The readiness of the body to respond to any eventuality exists as a level of *tone* or tension throughout the body. Tone describes the constant communication with all parts of the body which provides the capability to move and to survive. This calls for knowledge of the position of every muscle, joint and tendon. The ability to survive requires a perception of the internal and external environments. The pooling of the information about both provides an opportunity of interaction for the parts of the body we cannot reach in and touch. As active perceivers of the external environment, the feet and hands thus communicate with the internal environment.

Any sensory information gathered must be evaluated as a potential threat. For this reason, any sensory signal can be viewed as a stressor, demanding interaction with the body's tone. Thus, as a sensory organ, the feet and hands contribute to the body's tone. The contribution is made in the body's language of proprioception. Gathering information about movement are some very sophisticated gauges, such as deep pressure to the bottoms of the feet, the angulation of joints and the stretch of muscles and tendons.

In summary, because the hands and feet are sensory organs of locomotion, they have a special relationship with the body. Furthermore, because of the special relationship, they can serve as a means of interaction with the state of tension and energy consumption throughout the body.

THE BODY MANAGER:
TAKING ADVANTAGE OF THE WAY THE BODY WORKS

For every individual an opportunity exists to communicate with the whole body through the hands and feet. The special relationship between the feet, hands and body can be used for the purposes of:

- stress reduction
- energy savings
- building greater body awareness

The possibility for interaction becomes an opportunity for management when sensory experience is applied on a frequent and consistent basis. **The body manager is one who deliberately interacts with a part of his or her body, in this case hands and feet, to influence the whole body.** Such interaction allows one to manage the body's resources more efficiently and is at the very heart of the concept of "self help".

Energy

Energy is a body resource, a basis for the body economy. It exists always in limited supply, but there is a potential for regulation and an opportunity for conservation.

A certain amount of energy is required to move a certain distance. Each footstep can be seen as a unit of energy expended. Small savings on each footstep can add up to large gains. When one provides sensory experience to the hands and feet with this program, it helps break up the patterns of stress and allows one to begin to accrue savings and it makes it possible to apply these as investments in the body's total energy reserves. Energy-saving techniques for everyday activities may be applied to form a practical conservation program. So energy expended for tone or overall body communication may be influenced by applied sensory information.

Sensory Signals

Sensory signals provide a link of communication with the outside world and "local reporting" of information from the sensory organs which affects the body's economy. The sensing of the ground underfoot, such as in walking through sand, creates a demand on the whole body's economy and participates in the expenditure of the body's resources.

The application of consistent, frequent sensory stimulus creates a variety of signals which re-sets the body's tension level. In any learning situation, the more time a body spends "practicing" an event, the more proficient it becomes at it. The practice of variety lessens the demand on any one part of the body.

Locomotion

Locomotion is

- the expenditure of energy
- a sensory signal
- a participant in the body's readiness system

Tone

In terms of the body's economy, it is a major consumer of the body's resources. The possibility for interaction and for taking advantage of the way the body works exists because locomotion demands organization. The hands and feet are a part of the organization, the body's economy. They are a part of the body's

(1) energy consumption
(2) tension/tone level, and
(3) body awareness.

Tone budgets the expenditure of energy, taking into account past expenditures, present demands and future concerns. It is the active decision-making process involving these expenditures that is necessary to maintain readiness. Sleeping, for example, requires a state of readiness different from that of wakefulness.

Tone is an on-going changing process which is influenced by sensory signals, particularly those of locomotion.

The body manager uses interaction with the hands and feet on a frequent and consistent basis for the purposes of:

- energy savings
- stress reduction
- building greater body awareness.

PRINCIPLES OF BODY MANAGEMENT

1. It is possible to affect the body through sensory signals.

2. The feet and hands are sensory organs which gather information.

3. The primary information gathered is about locomotion (walking, running, standing).

4. Locomotion is part of the survival mechanism ensuring the ability to fight or flight.

5. Information about locomotion and internal organ function is pooled to ensure survival and to set a state of tension throughout the body on a day to day basis. Locomotion as an activity has a major influence on tension levels throughout the body.

6. Locomotion takes energy.

7. The consumption of energy for locomotion can contribute to "wear and tear" on the body.

8. As a learned activity, elements of locomotion can be practiced to become a more efficient activity which lessens the consumption of energy.

9. The elements of locomotion communicate through pressure, stretch and movement of joints, tendons and muscles.

10. It is possible to affect the body by mimicking the sensory signals of locomotion. The feet are of particular importance in the sensory/locomotor system. The frequent application of varied sensory signals to the hands and feet produces a cumulative effect, the net result of which is to break up patterns of stress, resetting energy consumption levels throughout the body and achieving a greater body awareness.

LEARNING THE BODY'S LANGUAGE

The body manager's role is to mimic some of the key sensory signals of the body in order to communicate with it. Our tools for the manager are reflexology, stride replication® and propriocise® . (Propriocise® will be fully discussed in other written work). These three fields of interest represent an organized application of key sensory signals to the hands and feet.

The key sensory signals are those of locomotion. To provide locomotive sensory information, proprioceptive sensations are mimicked. Proprioception is the body's self-perceiving mechanism, its picture of itself in motion. Reflexology, stride replication® and propriocise® merely practice proprioception.

Proprioception: The Language of Movement

The body's practice of proprioception actually begins at childhood and continues throughout life (see box). The stress placed on the body by walking and its sensory signals of proprioception establishes a pattern of tension throughout the body. Repeated exposure to stressors on a continuous basis produces "wear and tear". The repeated demands of walking over a lifetime can be a contributor to the gradual wearing down process known as aging.

Breaking the pattern of tension, however, can interrupt the cycle, providing a "vacation" from the usual routine. A program which mimics proprioception interrupts the usual pattern of tension by placing new and different demands on the body. An "exercise" of proprioception yields results appropriate to the way the body works. Improved adaptability, flexibility and a change in energy all result from the repeated interruption of tension. After all, repeated exercise improves muscle tone and circulation. Why then should the body not respond to the deliberate exercise of proprioception by improving its overall function in a similar manner?

The exercise of proprioception is the practice of its elements. Reports from muscles, tendons and joints are taken in the body's language of pressure and movement. An opportunity is thus provided to the individual to interact with the body in its own language.

BODY PERCEPTIONS

"Proprioceptive sensations are those that apprise the brain of the physical state of the body, including such sensations as (1) tension of the muscles, (2) tension of the tendons, (3) angulation of the joints, and (4) deep pressure from the bottom of the feet." Guyton, Arthur C., **Function of the Human Body,** W.B. Saunders Co., 1969, p. 272.

"Anyone who has watched an infant grow can appreciate the complexity of learning body positioning, especially in sitting, standing and walking. The waving of hands and feet in the newborn exhibits the beginning of a positioning awareness. The intricacies of sitting up are such that it takes two months for the infant to master it. Standing usually requires six months of experimentation, walking takes nine months, and bowel and bladder control take two years. Even at two years most infants have not perfected all of these tasks. The experimentation with possibilities of positions and movements can be seen throughout childhood. Tricycle and bicycle riding are ventures into balancing. Swinging on playground equipment, jumping rope, and other forms of what is considered 'play' are actually an educational process for the body. The awkward teenager is living testimony to the fact that this educational process is at least sixteen to eighteen years in duration." **Reflexions,** May/June, 1981, Vol. 2, No. 3.

"The positioning education of the body is a process of experimentation throughout childhood and even into the young adulthood ages of 18-20. An example of the body's learning process is practicing free throws in basketball. The first attempt may be far from the basket, but the body makes the gradual muscular adjustments to achieve the goal of putting the ball through the hoop. It is possible to consciously judge the ball as 'on target but too short' or 'long enough but off to the side'. But the actual means by which the body directs this muscle and that muscle to correct for 'off target' or 'too short' are unconscious and totally left up to the body's automatic positioning mechanism. It is this mechanism which receives its education in childhood.

What happens to this positioning mechanism in adulthood? The learning continues. The proprioceptive feedback is constantly provided and responded to. As we all know, however, the body response and performance is not quite the same in adulthood. That free throw is not accomplished with such ease at age 40 or 50 as it was at age 20 or even 30. Perhaps that crick in the neck does not allow ease of movement of the arm. Or perhaps the knee is not providing the spring it used to. What has happened?

The continuing education for body positioning in adults contains elements not present in childhood. In addition to the body's natural aging process, these elements include the body's experiences — that sprained ankle, the crick in the neck from sleeping on it wrong, the pain in the stomach. All of these experiences cause the body to hold itself differently. The tasks of walking, standing, and shooting basketballs are all modified by the body's experiences. That sprained ankle caused the body to make changes in its method of walking to minimize the amount of pain felt from the ankle. These changes range from the noticeable to the barely perceptible. The tightening of just a few muscle fibers, however, requires a corresponding shift in other fibers. The effect echoes throughout the body. The cumulative effect of the body's experiences on its positioning mechanism make the free throw a different event for the 20 year old body versus the 40 year old body." **Reflexions,** July/Aug, 1981, Vol. 2, No. 4.

The sensations which arise from muscle, joint and tendon are conveniently grouped under one heading not because of their anatomical source, but because they collaborate to provide the brain with a distinctive form of information. Sherrington called this 'proprioceptive sensation'. It tells the creature what it is doing and what is happening to it as a result of what it is doing: whether movements are going according to plan, or whether they are being obstructed. In other words, it monitors and refashions the creature's muscular enterprises from one moment to the next.

Without such information, there would be no knowing how one's limbs were arranged, and it would be impossible to find one's nose in the dark. The proprioceptive system supplies the brain with a coordinated map of all the available muscular resources and their current state of readiness." From **The Body in Question,** by Jonathan Miller. Copyright ©1978 by Jonathan Miller. Reprinted by permission of Random House, Inc.

". . . experiments have shown that exposure to . . . stressors can be withstood just so long. After the initial alarm reaction, the body becomes adapted and begins to resist, the length of the resistance period depending upon the body's innate adaptability and the intensity of the stressor. Yet, eventually exhaustion ensues.

We still do not know precisely just what is lost, except that it is not merely caloric energy, since food intake is normal during the stage of resistance. Hence, one would think that once adaptation has occurred, and energy is amply available, resistance should go on indefinitely. But just as an inanimate machine gradually wears out, even if it has enough fuel, so does the human machine sooner or later become the victim of constant wear and tear. These three stages are analogous to the three stages of man's life: childhood (with its characteristic low resistance and excessive responses to any kind of stimulus), adulthood (during which adaptation to most commonly encountered agents has occurred and resistance is increased) and finally, senility (characterized by irreversible loss of adaptability and eventual exhaustion) ending with death." **Stress Without Distress,** by Hans Selye, M.D. (J.B. Lippincott Co.) Copyright ©1974 by Hans Selye, M.D. Reprinted by permission of Harper & Row, Publishers, Inc.

Possibilities of Interaction: Working with Proprioception

The possibilities of interaction within the body's relationships lie in mimicking sensory signals. The signals of pressure and movement are the means by which we influence relationships.

To practice the sensory signals of proprioception on the hands and feet in an organized manner, the techniques of reflexology are applied on the basis of certain locomotive relationships.

Stride replication® is the practice of a variety of sensory signals applied on the basis of the locomotive responsibilities of the foot: weight-bearing and directional movement.

Self-help reflexology is the application of pressure to the hands and feet. Pressure may be applied to create either a stimulating effect or a deadening one. Alternating pressure is interpreted by the sensors of the body as a situation which demands additional information. The body attempts to "sense" a potential threat. The stimulation arises from the need for additional fuel, in the form of glucose and oxygen, demanded by the continuing evaluation of the on-going sensory stimulus.

Direct pressure is interpreted by the senses as a diminished need for information. The constancy of pressure poses no threat. The body evaluates direct pressure as a demand which is fixed and requires no further attention. Pain is one situation in which this situation would be desirable.

Our viewpoint is that the traditional definition of reflexology is actually a statement of observed effects. When reflexology techniques are viewed as the application of locomotive sensory signals, such effects would seem to be adequately explained. Locomotion and the body's state of readiness, tone, are inextricably linked.

"Foot reflexology is the study and practice of working reflexes in the feet which correspond to other parts of the body. With specific hand and finger techniques, reflexology causes responses (relaxation) in corresponding parts of the body. Relaxation is the first step to normalization, the body's return to a state of equilibrium or homeostasis, where circulation can flow unimpeded and supply nutrients and oxygen to the cells. With the restoration of homeostasis, the body's organs, which are actually aggregations of cells, may then return to a normal state or function as well."
Kunz & Kunz, **The Complete Guide to Foot Reflexology,**
Prentice-Hall Inc., 1982, p.2.

Using the Body's Relationships

The application of sensory information is based on certain locomotive relationships. In traditional reflexology, these relationships have been observed and noted. It is our contention that they are a reflection of the locomotive process. The demands of locomotion are such that these relationships form strong bonds.

The Body's Relationships

The locomotive relationships are the zonal, the reiterative and the referral. The strong bonds are formed by the demands of gravity, uprightness and the finely tuned organization of all body parts which are needed for walking.

In reflexology, reiterative relationships are the focus of the techniques. The zonal and referral relationships provide added emphasis to the reiterative. And when it is not possible to work with the hand or foot, the zonal and referral relationships provide an alternative.

The application of sensory information on the basis of locomotive sensations and relationships provides a variety of demands on the body. Thus the body is afforded an opportunity to view itself from a different perspective. The variety of stressors in the form of sensory signals provides relief from the wear and tear of constant stressors. The body has more information on which to make decisions, adjust to change and to act in a more integrated manner.

This description of adaptation notes the changing nature of tone, or normal operating state, in relationship to sensory signals. A consistant program of sensory signals results in a changed nature of tone. The body reflects what is practiced. Variety of stressor or sensory signal lessens the wear and tear on any one part.

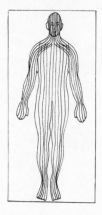

Zonal Relationships: Guidelines relating one part of the body to another.

The zonal relationship notes ten equal longitudinal segments running the length of the body which conveniently match the number of toes and fingers. The basic premise is that any part of one segment affects the entire segment. By extension, the application of sensory experience to any part of the segment affects the entire segment.

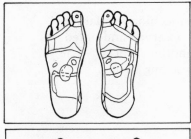

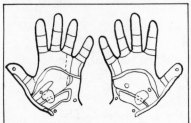

Reiterative Relationships: Mirroring the body whole on a body part.

Reiteration is a relationship in which the body whole is reflected on a body part. In reflexology, the body whole is reiterated on the hands and feet.

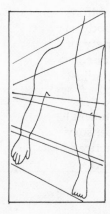

Referral Relationships: Relating the limbs using zones.

Referral relationships offer an additional manner in which to relate body parts, specifically the limbs. The relationship is based on zones. Following the basic premise, one segment of a zone affects and is affected by any other segment of the zone. Thus a segment of zone "one" in the arm relates to a segment of zone "one" in the leg.

A Locomotive View of the Relationships

Zonal relationships are a recognition that all body parts must move in relationship to gravity. Zones are a map of body parts in *relationship to gravity* while upright.

Reiteration maps the body parts in relationship to movement, it is a referral system of information necessary for movement.

"Reiteration is the body's systematic organizational scheme that establishes and maintains a communication throughout the body and thus ensures survival in a hostile environment."
Reflexions, Nov./Dec., 1982, Vol. 3, No. 6, p.5.

"In man, the nerve segments which together form the neck and arms are also the ones where the heart appears. The result is that the nerves bringing sensations from the heart are in the same segment as the nerves which bring sensation from the neck and arm. This relationship is preserved despite the fact that in the course of foetal development the heart migrates to a position which is quite remote from its original site . . . But the heart maintains its ancient parliamentary representation, despite its position in the body: the neck, arm, and upper chest continue to feel the pain for it. The same form of representation applies to all those parts which one would loosely call the 'innards'."
Jonathan Miller, *The Body in Question*, Random House, 1978, pp. 23-26.

The arms and legs must act in concert with each other to make walking a more efficient activity. Referral relationships relate the arms and legs using zones.

CHOOSING A PROGRAM OF WELLNESS: PUTTING TIME ON YOUR SIDE

The body manager deliberately uses sensory signals to interact with his or her own body. Consistency and frequent application is needed because of the way the body works. Basically, it learns what it practices. Interruption of tension on a frequent basis acts to teach the body that a different level of operating tension is possible.

Furthermore, with frequency of application, the sensory signals create a self-rewarding effect. The variety provides a rest and change of pace for the system. The contrast between what the feet and hands feel like before and after being worked on motivates one to continue.

Eventually the application of sensory signals will become second nature. The idea is to conveniently fit the techniques into the daily schedule. Factors to consider are the time available and finding a technique for the time and place.

There are ways to create time. You can do other things and still work on yourself. There is much possible free time, such as when riding in a car as a passenger, while watching television, while visiting with friends, or while talking on the phone. Keeping a foot roller at the dining room table makes it convenient for use while sipping coffee or talking after meals. Evaluate your schedule and discover what time you can create.

Set up specific times during the day for specific activities. Foot rolling can be done at the breakfast table, hand work on the way to work, for example. Make it a habit and you will find yourself doing it almost unconsciously. For further information see "Time Planning for Consistency."

TIME PLANNING FOR CONSISTENCY

Sensory signal techniques can be applied in a few seconds or over a period of time. To fit application of techniques into your daily schedule, use this chart to consider available time. Tie your program into something you do regularly, such as watching the evening news on television.

Time Available	Finding Time	Places Where Time Is Available
Very limited	At a stop light In a traffic jam	Car
A few minutes	Commuting (passenger) Commuting Waiting Coffee break	Car Bus, train, plane For an appointment
More time	Gatherings	Meeting Sporting event theater
More time	While doing paperwork Reading the newspaper	At the office At the dining table
Extended time	While watching TV In the tub Visiting with friends	Easy chair

FINDING A TECHNIQUE FOR THE TIME AND PLACE

Not all techniques are appropriate to be applied at all times. It may not always be appropriate to remove one's shoes to work on feet, for example.

Technique features	Hand	Foot
Any time / any place Easy to learn / easy to do	The grip techniques	Rotating on a point
Easy to learn / easy to do	Golf ball techniques	Foot roller technique
Not every place		Golf ball techniques
Moderate learning not every place	Thumb & finger walking	Thumb & finger walking
Easy to learn / easy to do not every place	Directional movement	Stride replication®

STARTING UP YOUR PROGRAM

STARTING OFF

1.   Pick a starting point, choose an area of interest. Refer to "Special Interests" and/or "Body Parts" for information about patterns relating to the area of interest. Start with a limited number of specific techniques which fit conveniently into the daily schedule. An over-burdening, inconvenient program will be hard to stick with.

2.   Select techniques appropriate to you. See "Finding a Technique for Time and Place". See "Techniques". The chapter includes easy-to-learn, quickly applied techniques as well as techniques which can be developed.

3.   Make a rough plan of when to apply the techniques. See "Time Planning for Consistency." In planing, think in terms of your day. If your time is limited, plan around that factor. If you have more time available, your plan may reflect that as a factor.

4.   Get started. Work with the area of interest daily according to your time available. Consider a whole hand and/or foot workout once or twice a week. At the end of a week, review your program. By this time, some techniques may or may not fit naturally into your day. Re-evaluate the time available and appropriate techniques.

     If you should happen to miss a day here or there, just go back to your program the next day. If you find that you are missing more days than not, or if you don't seem to follow your program completely every day, review your program and your goals. Have you chosen too ambitious a program with too many areas and not enough time in your day to work them? Are you just discouraged with your lack of progress? For encouragement declare a break in your program and give yourself time to re-assess your goals and your available time. During your week's re-assessment, pick one area to work. The results in that one area should give you the incentive to go on.

DEVELOPING A CONSISTENT PATTERN

The sensory signal techniques are self-rewarding. The cumulative effect of their application calls for further exploration. This might mean the addition of a technique to work a given area or finding a new area of interest.

To further explore an area of interest, consider other techniques relevant to the area. For example, to a program of grip techniques, add thumb and finger walking techniques for variety.

Accomplishment in working with one area leads to the selection of a new one. See "Special Interests" and "Body Parts." The original area can still be worked with. To spend less time with it, choose a quick and easy technique.

QUESTIONS AND ANSWERS

Q. **How long should I work on my hands and feet?**

A. This is a matter of individual choice. Consistency is the important thing. Working five minutes every day, for example, is preferrable to occasional work for twenty minutes.

Q. **How often should I work on my hands and feet?**

A. Note the affects of the technique applications and then gauge your work accordingly.

Q. **How long will it take to get results? What kind of results can I expect?**

A. The length of time needed to achieve results is an individual matter. One thought to keep in mind is that the effects begin upon the application of sensory signals. Results are the accumulation of the effects of applying sensory signals. The more time one spends applying the techniques, the more results will be possible.

Q. **Which is better, working on feet or working on hands?**

A. Both have their unique qualities. The hands have the advantage of accessibility. The impact of sensory signals on the feet is perhaps greater as the feet are the more neglected of the two sensory organs.

Q. **What can reflexology tell me about my health?**

A. Reflexology is an assessment in the body's terms. These are not the same terms as those developed by medical science for diagnosis. Reflexology provides an assessment of the self-perceiving mechanism of the body.

Q. **Which is better, reflexology work done by a practitioner or done by myself?**

A. The work of a practitioner has its benefits. The body's perspective of sensory signals as applied by a practitioner is different than that of self application. A talented foot worker provides relaxation unavailable through self-application. The services of a practitioner are another investment in a program of wellness.

On the other hand, whether or not you have access to a practitioner, a sensory signal is a sensory signal no matter who applies it. Self application is always a valid approach.

Q. **I don't seem to have the energy to get started working on my hands and feet. What should I do?**

A. Start a cycle of relaxation. Look at the techniques in this book and find one to begin with. Use it to build consistency. This will provide cumulative effects needed to develop a more ambitious program. Never force yourself to follow a rigid program. Find the energy through finding techniques which appeal to you.

Q. **I'm not getting results. What should I do?**
A. Try a change in program.
   Try a different technique.
   Work for a longer time.

Q. **I've hit a plateau and don't seem to be making progress. What should I do?**
A. Integration of new information by the body requires time. There are two approaches. One is to add techniques related to the special interest. The other is to maintain a program of moderate effort. It is a matter of personal preference.

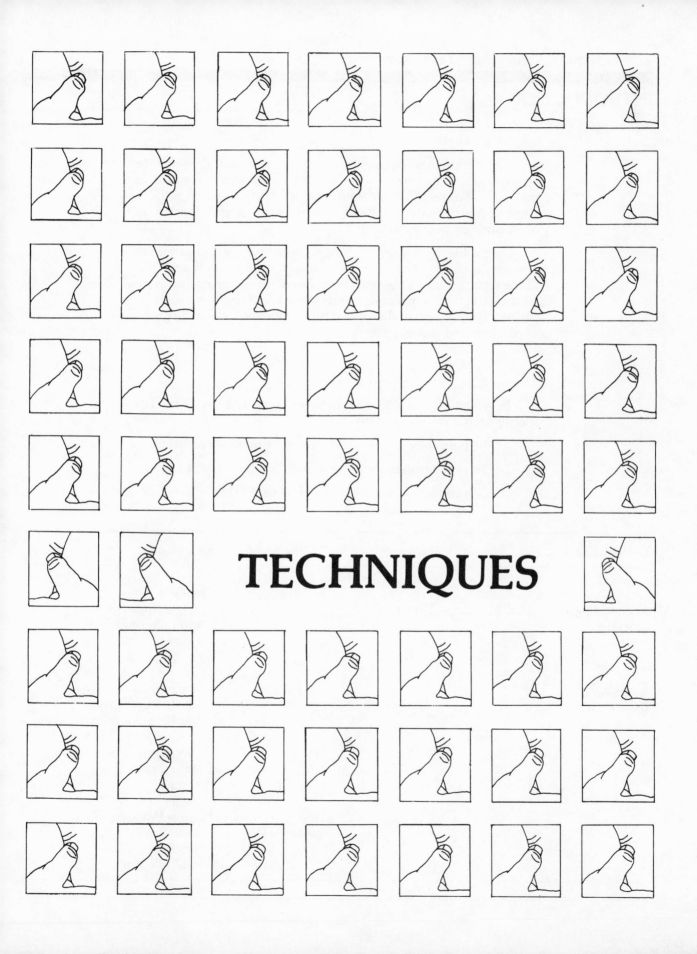

TECHNIQUES

INTRODUCTION

The techniques detailed in this chapter are designed to organize and refine the application of pressure and movement to the hands and feet. The system utilizes the body's natural skills to target various parts of the hand or foot to reduce spot tension by using pressure and movement.

Reflexology is the practice of sensory experience, primarily pressure, applied precisely to specific parts of the hands and feet. Stride replication® is the practice of key sensory signals necessary for walking. The complex demands made on the body by such experience form a kind of dialogue with the body in its own language of pressure and movement.

In *reflexology*, a digit exerts pressure to a target area. The specific technique is based on:

- the point of contact desired for spot tension reduction
- the type of pressure to be exerted for the desired effect
- the surface of the foot or hand to be worked.

Desired Effect	Pressure	Technique

Deadening (pain-killing, blocking)	Direct	The Grip
		  single finger grip
		  multiple finger grip
		the pinch
		direct grip

Stimulating (educating)	Alternating	The Grip
		  single finger grip
		  multiple finger grip
		  the pinch
		  direct grip
		Rotating on a Point
		  thumb
		  finger
		Thumb Walking
		  thumb
		  finger
		  multiple finger

In *stride replication*®, movement of the hand and foot is specifically practiced. The specific technique is based on:

- the type of movement to be mimicked for the desired effect
- the portion of the hand or foot to be worked for spot tension reduction.

Desired Effect	Movement	Technique
Practice of movement	Locomotive	
	(1) Directional movement of the foot	Varying sensory signal
Education		Varying weight bearing
	(2) Weight bearing	Directional movement
Relaxation	responsibilities	of foot

A Note on Handedness

Practice using both hands as working hands. (DO NOT become a single-handed reflexologist.) It may be awkward (at first) for a right-handed person to use the left hand as a working hand and vice versa. Keep in mind that both the working hand and the hand or foot being worked are receiving benefits.

REFLEXOLOGY

Three Basic Techniques

THE GRASP: A TECHNIQUE FUNDAMENTAL

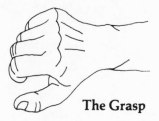

The Grasp

The basis of the reflexology techniques is a grasp. In its simplest form, the grasp is used by an infant to grab onto an offered finger.

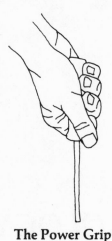

The Power Grip

In everyday life, we use the grasp to turn a screw driver. This is a *power grip,* used when strength is needed. The thumb reinforces the efforts of the fingers.

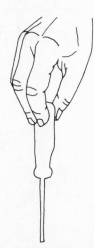

The Precision Grip

The *precision grip* is used when fine touch is needed. The thumb works in opposition to the fingers for accuracy and delicacy of touch.

In this section the grasp (variations of the *power grip* and *precision grip* is used most effectively to apply sensory experience to specific parts of the hands and feet.

THE GRIP TECHNIQUE

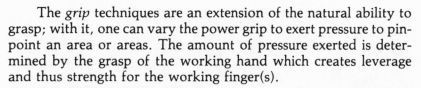

The *grip* techniques are an extension of the natural ability to grasp; with it, one can vary the power grip to exert pressure to pinpoint an area or areas. The amount of pressure exerted is determined by the grasp of the working hand which creates leverage and thus strength for the working finger(s).

Fingernail marks may be a problem in the grip techniques as a whole. Be aware of the fingernail marks you may be leaving. If you are concerned about nail marks or if you have long nails, use the flat of the finger or thumb to exert pressure, or consider the use of the eraser end of a pencil.

The finger or thumb tip is the point of contact for the pressure.

In the *single finger/multiple finger grip* techniques, the thumb and palm of the hand reinforces the efforts of the fingers by acting as a brace when the finger tip is the point of contact for the pressure.

In the *pinch grip*, the flats of the thumb and finger serve both as a point of contact and brace.

In the *direct grip*, the flat of the thumb is the point of contact and fingers serve as a brace.

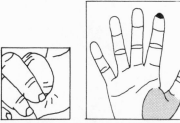

Single Finger Grip

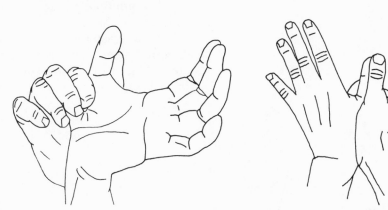

The *single finger* grip technique is used to pinpoint areas of the hand or foot. To practice the *single finger* grip technique, grasp the hand as shown. The palm of the working hand rests on top of the hand being worked. The tip of the finger is placed on the area to be worked. The palm acts with a bracing effect and the tip of the finger makes contact to exert pressure.

(continued on next page)

THE GRIP TECHNIQUE

(continued from preceding page)

To create alternating pressure:

- exert pressure repeatedly with the finger tip
- move the hand being worked
- move the entire working hand or
- any combination of two of the elements listed.

To create direct pressure:

- exert pressure with the finger tip for 15 to 30 seconds.

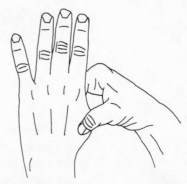

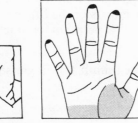

Multiple Finger Grip

The *multiple finger grip* technique is used to cover broader areas of the hand or foot. To practice the *multiple finger grip* technique, grasp the hand as shown. Make contact with the tips of all four fingers. The palm acts with a bracing effect. To create alternating or direct pressure, see the steps outlined for the *single finger grip.*

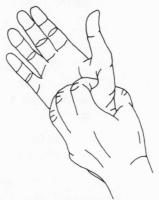

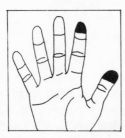

Pinch Grip

The opposition of the thumb and finger is used to exert pressure in the webbing of the hand or foot. The flats of the thumb and finger serve both as a point of contact and brace.

To practice the technique on the hand, the flats of the thumb and finger are placed on the top and palm of the hand in the webbing. The finger serves as backing while the thumb exerts most of the pressure. Be aware of fingernails.

To create direct pressure: Pinch the flesh of the webbing of the hand between the thumb and finger. Exert the amount of pressure desired for 15 to 30 seconds.

To create alternating pressure: Pinch the flesh of the webbing of the hand between the thumb and finger. Bend and unbend the first joint of the thumb to create an alternating pressure. Place the thumb and finger in the webbing of the hand. Use the *thumb walking* technique to create alternating pressure.

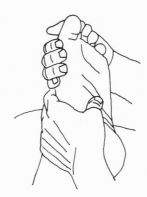

Direct Grip

Direct or alternating pressure is created by the flat of the thumb of the working hand and movement of the foot by the holding hand. To practice the *direct grip* technique, place the flat of the thumb on the bottom of the foot. The holding hand grasps the foot with the palm of the hand resting on top of the foot and the fingers wrapped around the inside edge of the foot. Movement is created by pushing with the heel of the hand on the top of the foot. The working hand is in position for the *thumb walking* technique but the thumb remains in a stationary position. In this position, pressure is exerted by the flat of the thumb and the amount of pressure varies with the movement of the heel of the hand.

To create direct pressure: Position the hands on the foot. Push with the heel of the hand to move the foot. The flat of the thumb exerts pressure. Exert the amount of pressure desired for the length of time desired.

To create alternating pressure: Maintain the thumb in a stationary position. Use the heel of the hand to move the foot up and down, thus creating an alternating pressure.

ROTATING ON A POINT TECHNIQUE

The *rotating on a point* technique is the ultimate example of how to get maximum results with minimum effort. It is a multi-purpose technique, and it can be used to increase flexibility of the foot. Leverage combined with pinpoint pressure by the thumb or finger are crucial to the effectiveness of this technique. Simply stated, the technique is one of pinpointing an area and rotating the ankle, thus the term "rotating on a point".

The finger is most effective pinpointing the areas on top of the foot and to the outside. Here the thumb provides the leverage. The thumb is most effective in pinpointing areas on the sides of the foot with the fingers providing the necessary leverage.

The *rotating on a point* technique exerts pressure using the grasp of the hand and the flat of the thumb or finger(s) in the power grip. A turning of the foot or hand being worked creates alternating pressure.

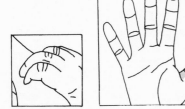
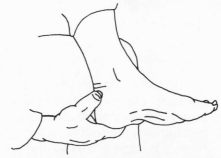

Finger Rotating on a Point

To practice the finger *rotating on a point* technique, grasp the foot as shown. The grasp of the hand braces the finger. The flat of the finger serves as point of contact. Place the flat of the finger on the area to be worked. Rotate the foot in a clockwise direction and then a counter-clockwise direction. Re-position the finger of the working hand and repeat.

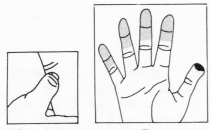

Thumb Rotating on a Point

To practice the thumb *rotating on a point* technique, grasp the foot. The grasp of the hand braces the thumb. The flat of the thumb serves as point of contact. Position the flat of the thumb on the area to be worked. Note that the positioning of the thumb requires that the heel of the working hand be lifted from the surface of the ankle. The hand arches between the fingers and the flat of the thumb, opening up a space between the foot and hand. The opposition of the thumb and the fingers creates the leverage for the pressure exerted by the thumb. The pull of the fingers varies the pressure exerted.

Apply pressure with the flat of the thumb. Rotate the foot in a clockwise direction and then a counter-clockwise direction, drawing circles in the air with the big toe.

THUMB AND FINGER WALKING TECHNIQUE

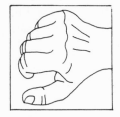

The goal of the *thumb* and *finger walking* techniques is to exert a constant steady pressure while contouring to the surfaces of the hands and feet. The interplay of the fingers and thumb provide the ability to contour and exert pressure to a variety of surfaces.

A Lesson in Thumb Walking

The *thumb walking* technique features qualities of both the precision and the power grips. The fingers act in unison to grasp, while the thumb is free to provide pressure in opposition in a very precise manner. The tip of the thumb is the point of contact for the exertion of pressure. The natural angle of the thumb is such that the outside edge works optimally in opposition to the fingers to create pressure.

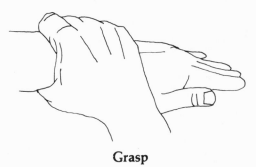

Grasp

To practice the *thumb walking* technique, first imagine reaching up to grasp a chin-up bar. The hands are in an open grasp with the fingers holding on.

Grasp: Grasp the arm.

Lift off: Unwrap the thumb from the grasp. Maintain the grasp of the fingers.

Contact: *Place the tip of the thumb on the surface* of the arm. The outside edge is the point of contact. The fingertips maintain the grasp. The hand arcs between the fingertips and the edge of the thumb, creating an open space between the hand and arm. A downward pressure exerted by the thumb tip is thus created. The pressure varies with the tension created between the thumb and fingers. An increase of pull by the fingers by lowering the wrist increases the pressure exerted by the thumb tip.

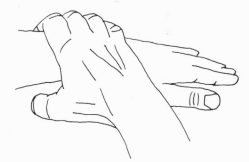

Lift Off

With the thumb tip on the surface of the arm, and the thumb held straight, drop the wrist. Note the increased pressure by the thumb tip.

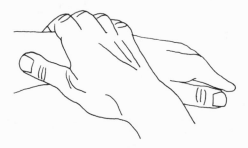

Contact
(continued on next page)

(continued from preceding page)

The object of the *thumb walking* technique is to exert a constant, steady pressure with the thumb tip. The entire hand participates in this technique but the first joint of the thumb is the only moving part. The first joint bends and unbends to move the thumb tip in a forward direction. The second joint of the thumb does not move. It participates in the creation of leverage and, thus, pressure.

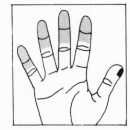

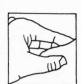

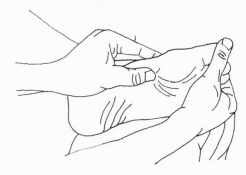

To practice the *thumb walking* technique on the foot, grasp the foot and hold it back. With the working hand, grasp the foot. The fingers rest on top of the foot and serve as an anchor, bracing the thumb. The outside edge of the thumb is the point of contact on the bottom of the foot.

Now practice walking with the thumb on the bottom of the foot. Move only the first joint of the thumb. Any change of pressure is a result of tightening the grasp of the fingers and thumb. When the grasp is tightened, the wrist is lowered.

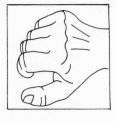

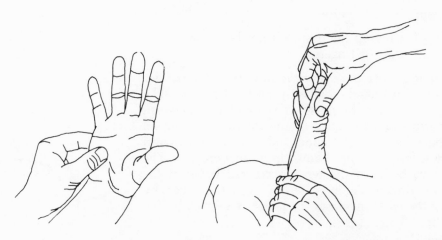

The *thumb walking* technique is the exertion of pressure while contouring to the surfaces of the feet and hands. The interplay between the fingers and the thumb provides the ability to contour to the many different surfaces.

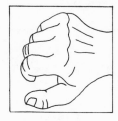

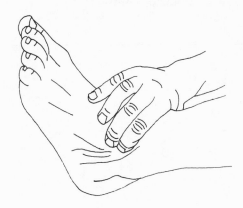

 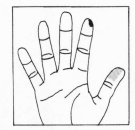

Single Finger Walking

To practice the *single finger walking* technique, first grasp the ankle. Lift the fingers from the ankle and draw them back so that the tip of the index finger rests on the ankle. As in the *thumb walking* technique, the pressure applied by the finger tip is created by the tension between the thumb and the finger. Again, the object of the *finger walking* technique is to create a constant steady pressure. The first joint of the finger bends and unbends to move the finger forward.

 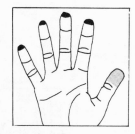

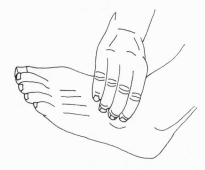

Multiple Finger Walking

To practice the *multiple finger walking* technique, grasp the ankle. Lift the fingers and draw them back so that the tips of the fingers rest on the ankle. The thumb acts as a brace as the fingers move forward.

TECHNIQUE SUMMARY CHART: THREE BASIC TECHNIQUES

Technique	Point of Contact/ Brace	Parts of Hand Worked By

I. The Grip

Single Finger

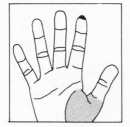
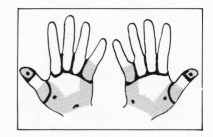

Multiple Finger

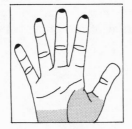
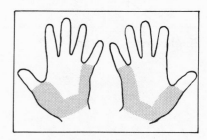

The Pinch

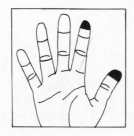
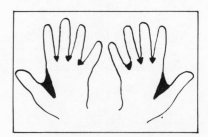

Parts of Foot
Worked By

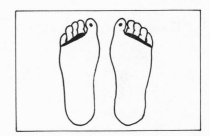

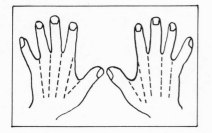

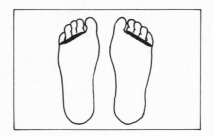

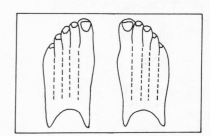

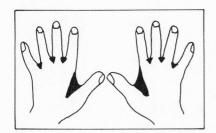

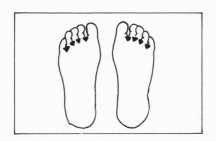

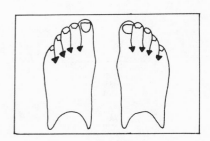

TECHNIQUE SUMMARY CHART: THREE BASIC TECHNIQUES

Technique	Point of Contact/ Brace	Parts of Hand Worked By

Direct Grip

 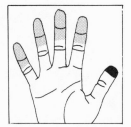 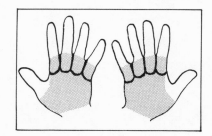

II. Rotating on a Point

Finger

 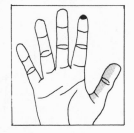 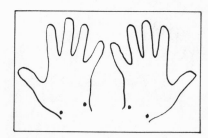

Thumb

 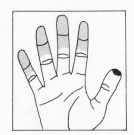 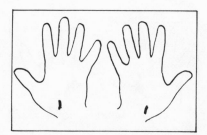

Parts of Foot
Worked By

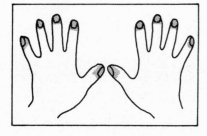

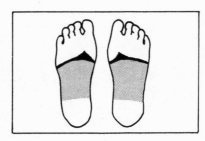

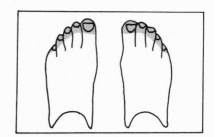

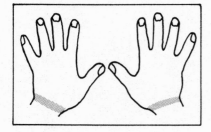

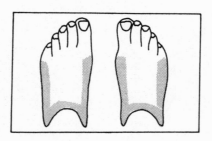

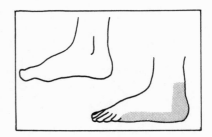

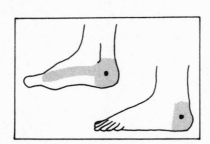

TECHNIQUE SUMMARY CHART: THREE BASIC TECHNIQUES

Technique	Point of Contact/ Brace	Parts of Hand Worked By

III. Thumb Walking / Finger Walking

Thumb Walking

 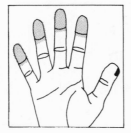 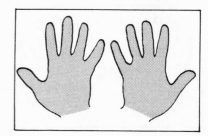

Finger Walking

 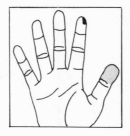 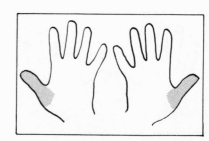

Multiple
Finger Walking

 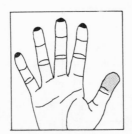 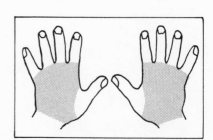

Parts of Foot
Worked By

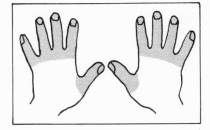

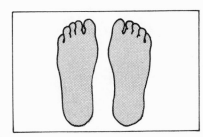

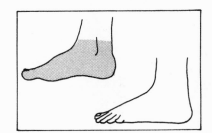

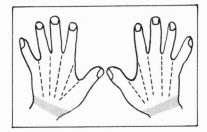

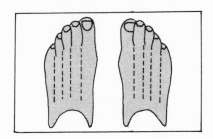

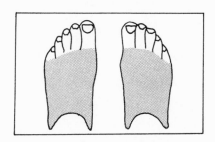

FOOT REFLEXOLOGY

Applied Techniques

BOTTOM OF FOOT: Thumb Walking

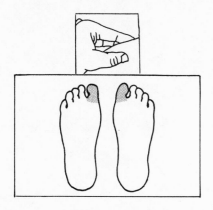

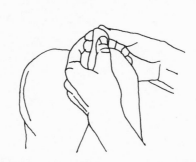

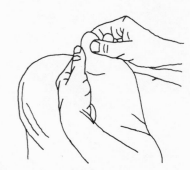

Place the fingers of the holding hand on top of the foot. Use the holding hand to support the toe. Rest the fingers of the working hand on top of the fingers of the holding hand. Position the working thumb and use the *thumb walking* technique to walk up the toe. Make several passes.

Variation: ⟶ ⟵

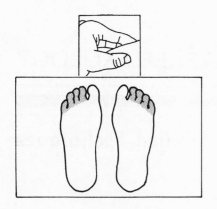

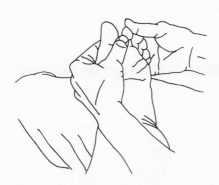

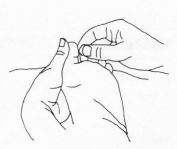

Place the fingers of the holding hand on top of the foot. Use the holding hand to support the toes and to minimize movement. Rest the fingers of the working hand on top of the fingers of the holding hand. Position the working thumb at the base of the toe. Use the *thumb walking* technique to walk up the toe. Re-position the thumb and in successive passes, cover the center and side of the toe.

Variation: ⟶ ⟵

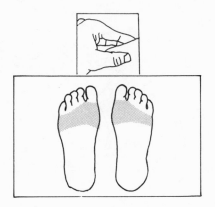

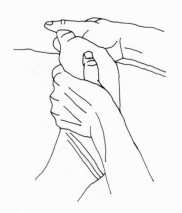

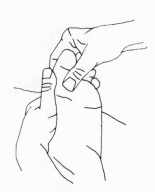

Hold the foot back with the holding hand. Place the thumb in the trough between the big toe and second toe. Use the *thumb walking* technique to walk up the trough. Re-position the working hand and work through each trough.

Switch hands. The holding hand becomes the working hand and vice versa. Use the thumb walking technique to walk up each trough beginning with the trough to the outside of the foot.

Variation: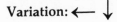

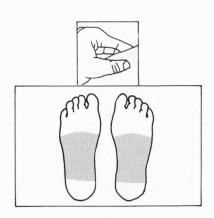

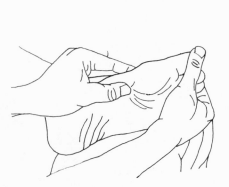

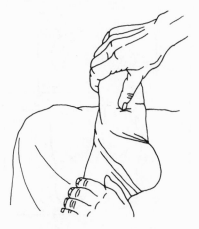

Hold the foot back. Note the tendon on the bottom of the foot. It serves as a guideline. Place the thumb of the working hand to the inside edge of the foot. Use the *thumb walking* technique to walk up the foot along the tendon. Re-position the thumb and use the *thumb walking* technique to walk across the foot. Make successive passes to work the area.

Variation: ⟶ ↓

BOTTOM OF FOOT: Grip Techniques

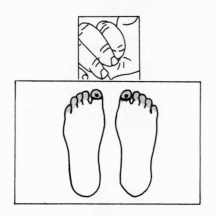

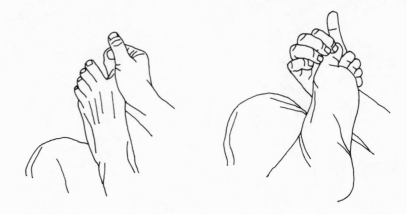

Place the palm of the hand on top of the foot as shown. Rest the finger tip on the area of the big toe on the bottom of the foot to be worked. Using the *single finger grip* technique, exert an alternating pressure.

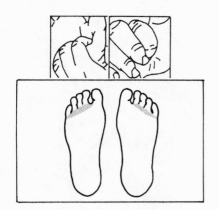

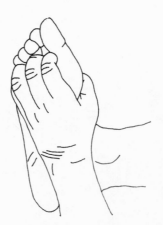

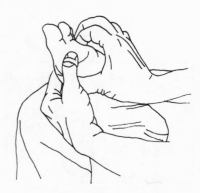

Place the tips of the fingers on the ledge formed across the base of the toes. The hand grasps the foot and wraps around to provide leverage. Using the *multiple finger grip* technique, grip with the fingers in a downward direction. Be careful of fingernails.

Variation: A *single finger grip* technique may be used to work closer to the base of each toe.

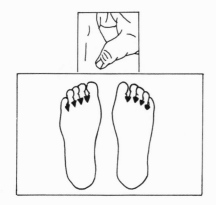

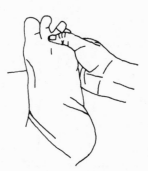

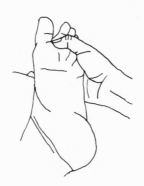

Place the thumb on the bottom of the foot to be worked. The fingers rest on the top of the foot and serve as a backstop. Use the *thumb walking* technique to work the webbing between the toes. Work as far into the trough as the padding on the ball of the foot will allow. Be careful not to work too deeply into the soft skin between the toes.

Variation: Pinch the thumb and forefinger together to exert alternating pressure to the area. Re-position and repeat.

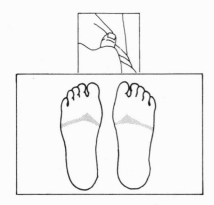

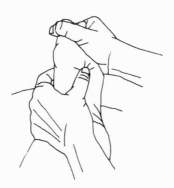

To use the *direct grip* technique, grasp the foot with the holding hand. Place the flat of the thumb of the working hand on the bottom of the foot in the area to be worked. With the holding hand, rotate the foot, moving against the stationary thumb of the working hand.

(continued on next page)

(continued from preceding page)

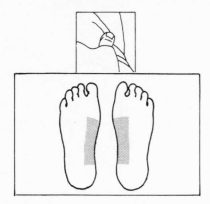

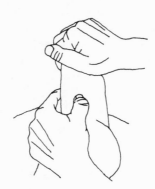

To use the *direct grip* technique, grasp the foot with the holding hand. The palm rests on top of the foot and the fingers wrap around the inside edge. Place the flat of the thumb of the working hand on the bottom of the foot in the area to be worked. The working thumb remains stationary as the holding hand moves the foot to create an alternating pressure at the point of contact. Using the heel of the holding hand, move the foot so that the outside edge of the foot is moved towards you.

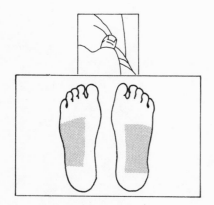

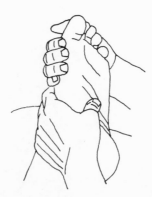

To use the *direct grip* technique, grasp the joint below the big toe with the holding hand. Place the flat of the thumb of the working hand on the bottom of the foot in the area to be worked. With the holding hand, bend the foot towards you. The thumb of the working hand remains stationary as pressure is exerted at the point of contact by movement of the foot.

TOP OF FOOT: Miscellaneous Techniques

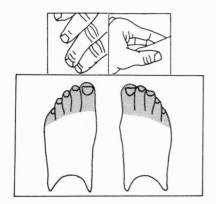

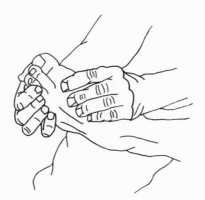

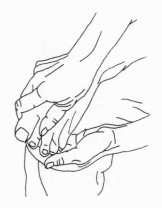

Place the finger of the working hand on the toe to be worked. Use the *finger walking* technique to walk across the toe. Experiment with each of the possible directions;
Cover the nails and the base of the toe.

Variation: To use the *thumb walking* technique, place the fingers on the bottom of the foot to provide leverage. Place the thumb at the base of the nail. Use the inside corner of the thumb to exert pressure. Re-position and re-apply pressure.

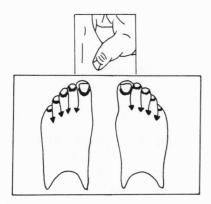

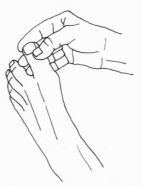

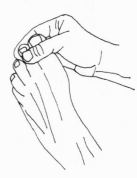

Rest the toe between the fingers and thumb. Using the *pinch grip* technique, bring the fingers and thumb together. The corner of the thumb exerts pressure to the top of the toe.

Rest the foot between the fingers and thumb. Use the *pinch grip* technique to exert pressure to the webbing between the toes.

(continued on next page)

(continued from preceding page)

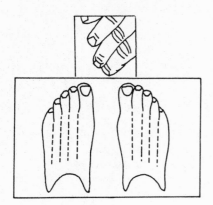

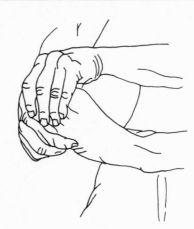

Use the holding hand to separate the big toe and second toe. The trough between the toes is thus accentuated. Place the finger of the working hand at the base of the toe. Use the *finger walking* technique to walk down the side of trough to the inside of the foot.

Switch hands. The holding hand becomes the working hand and vice versa. Work as above using the *finger walking* technique to walk down the side of the trough to the outside of the foot.

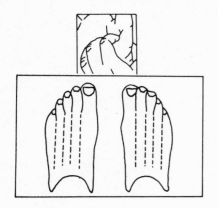

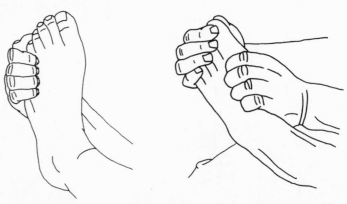

Place the fingers of the working hand in the trough formed by the first and second toes on top of the foot. Use the *multiple finger grip* technique to exert pressure to the inside of the trough. Re-position the working hand and work another part of the trough.

Re-position the working hand and work each trough.

Switch hands. The opposite hand is now the working hand. Use the *multiple finger grip* technique to exert pressure to the side of the trough toward the outside of the foot.

Variation: Use the holding hand to rotate the foot against the fingertips of the working hand on top of the foot.

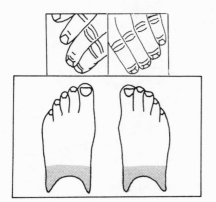

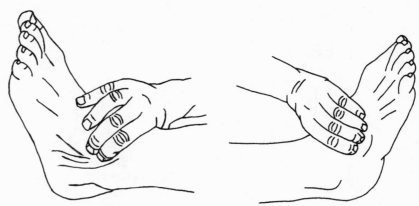

Place the finger of the working hand on top of the foot. The thumb is placed on the bottom of the foot to provide leverage. Use the *multiple finger walking* technique to walk across the foot. Reposition the working hand and walk across the area in successive passes.

Variation: *Finger walking* technique.

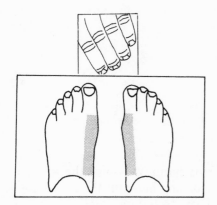

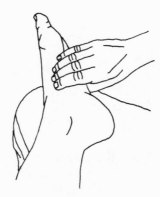

Place the thumb of the working hand on the outside edge of the foot. Rest the fingers of the working hand on the inside edge of the foot. Use the *multiple finger walking* technique to walk around the edge of the foot.

SIDE OF FOOT, INSIDE: Thumb Walking

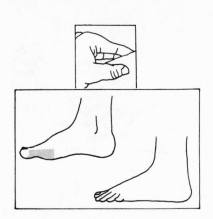

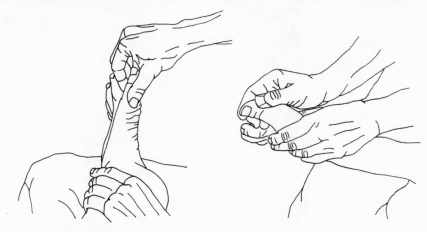

Place the fingers of the working hand on the side of the big toe. Place the thumb of the working hand on the opposite side of the toe. Use the *thumb walking* technique to walk down the inside edge of the foot.

Variation: Pull with the fingers to create additional leverage. Use the *thumb walking* technique to walk down the inside edge of the foot.

Variation: ←

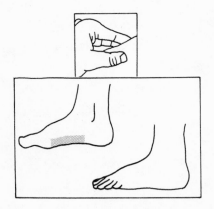

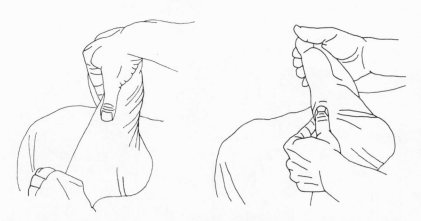

Place the fingers of the working hand on top of the foot for leverage. Place the thumb of the working hand on the inside edge of the foot. Using the *thumb walking* technique, walk down the edge of the foot. Make several passes.

Variation: Use the *thumb walking* technique to walk up the inside edge of the foot. The holding hand steadies the foot. The fingers of the working hand are placed on top of the foot for leverage.

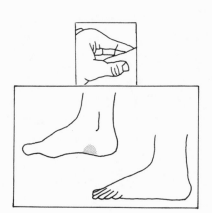

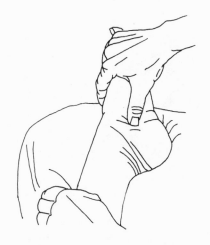

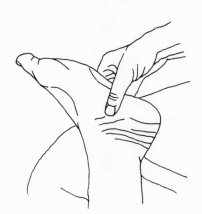

The fingers of the working hand rest on top of the foot to provide leverage. Use the *thumb walking* technique to walk down the foot. Make several passes.

Variation: ←

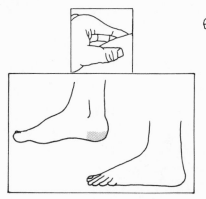

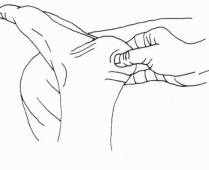

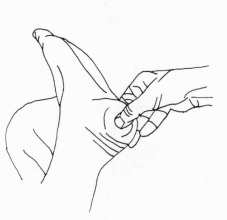

Rest the fingers of the working hand under the heel of the foot for leverage. Use the *thumb walking* technique to walk up the edge of the heel.

Variation: ←

SIDE OF FOOT, OUTSIDE: Finger Walking/Rotating on a Point

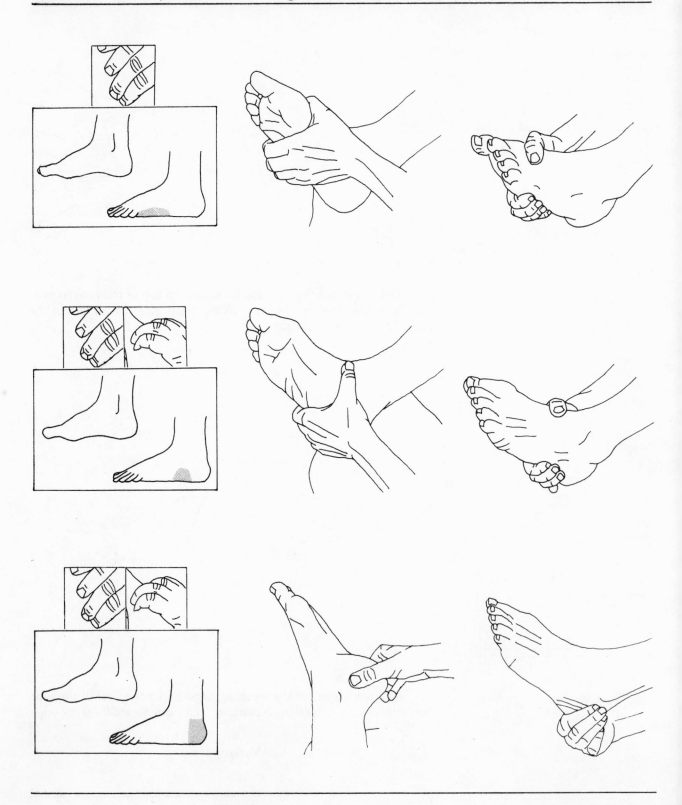

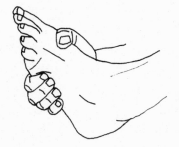

Grasp the foot. Rest the thumb of the working hand on the inside edge of the foot for leverage. Place the finger on the outside edge of the foot. Use the *finger walking* technique to walk around the outside edge of the foot.

Variation: As above, *rotating on a point, multiple finger walking.*

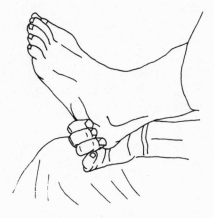

Grasp the foot. Rest the thumb of the working hand on the inside edge of the foot for leverage. Place the finger on the outside edge of the foot. Use the *finger walking* technique to walk around the outside edge of the foot.

Variation: As above, *rotating on a point, multiple finger walking.*

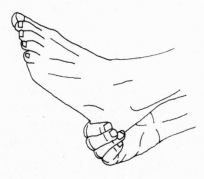

Grasp the foot. Rest the thumb of the working hand on the inside edge of the foot for leverage. Place the finger on the outside edge of the foot. Use the *finger walking* technique to walk around the outside edge of the foot.

Variation: As above, *rotating on a point, multiple finger walking.*

SIDE OF FOOT, INSIDE: Rotating on a Point

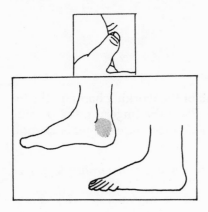

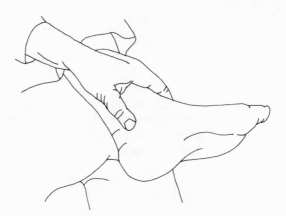

Grasp the foot. To use this *rotating on a point* technique, exert pressure with the flat of the thumb. Draw circles in the air with the big toe, rotating the foot first in a clockwise direction, then a counter-clockwise direction. Re-position the thumb and repeat. Vary the pressure by pulling against the fingers.

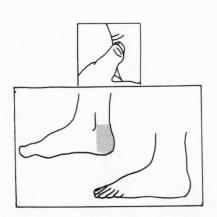

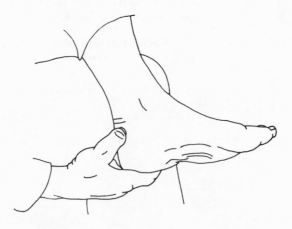

Rest the heel of the foot on the fingers. To use this *rotating on a point* technique, exert pressure with the corner of the thumb. Turn the foot first in a clockise direction and then a counter-clockwise direction. Re-position the thumb and repeat. Tighten or loosen the grasp to vary pressure.

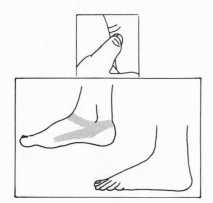

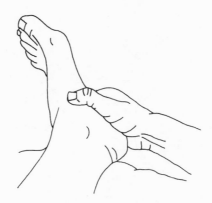

Grasp the foot. To use this *rotating on a point* technique, exert pressure with the corner of the thumb. Rotate the foot first in a clockwise direction, then a counter-clockwise direction. Re-position the thumb and repeat. Tighten or loosen the grasp to vary pressure.

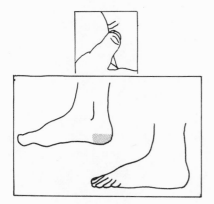

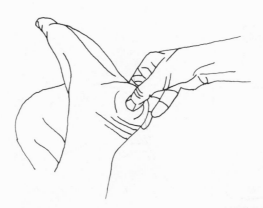

Rest the heel of the foot on the fingers. To use this *rotating on a point* technique, use the corner of the thumb to exert pressure. Rotate the foot first in a clockwise direction and then a counter-clockwise direction. Re-position the thumb and repeat. Tighten or loosen the grasp to vary pressure.

SIDE OF FOOT, INSIDE/OUTSIDE: Rotating on a Point

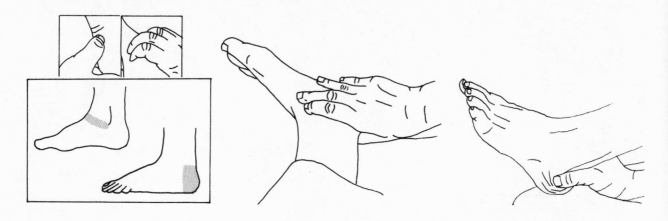

Grasp the foot. In this *rotating on a point* technique, use both the finger tip and corner of the thumb to exert pressure. Turn the foot first in a clockwise direction, then a counter-clockwise direction. Re-position the thumb and repeat. Tighten or loosen the grasp to vary pressure.

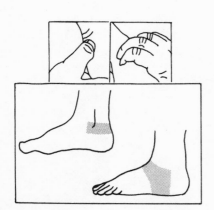

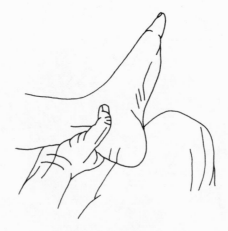

Grasp the foot. In this *rotating on a point* technique, use both the finger tip and corner of the thumb to exert pressure. Turn the foot first in a clockwise direction and then a counter-clockwise direction. Reposition the thumb and repeat. Tighten or loosen the grasp to vary pressure.

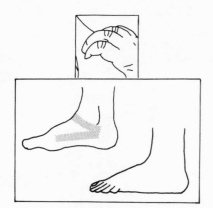

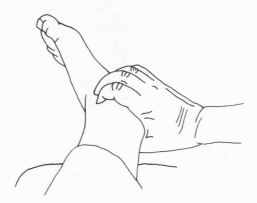

Grasp the foot. To use this *rotating on a point* technique, exert pressure with the finger tip. Draw circles in the air with the big toe, rotating the foot first in a clockwise direction and then a counter-clockwise direction. Re-position the finger and repeat. Tighten or loosen the grasp to vary pressure.

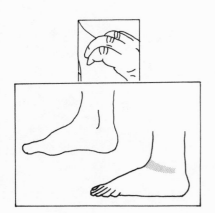

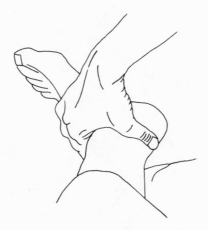

Grasp the foot. To use this *rotating on a point* technique, exert pressure with the finger tip. Turn the foot first in a clockwise direction, then a counter-clockwise direction. Re-position the finger and repeat. Tighten or loosen the grasp to vary pressure.

SIDE OF FOOT, INSIDE: Golf Ball

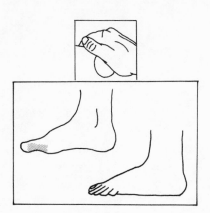

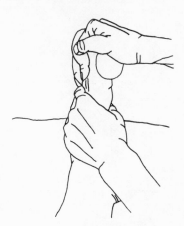

Note: *Be aware of your individual response to the pressure exerted by the hard surface of the golf ball. Choose a level of pressure according to your preference and comfort level.*

Cup the golf ball in the working hand. The big toe is trapped between the fingers of the working hand and the golf ball. Roll the edge of the toe with the golf ball. Make several passes. Pressure varies by tightening the grasp of the working hand.

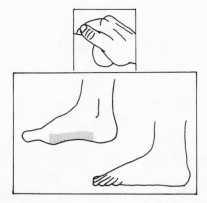

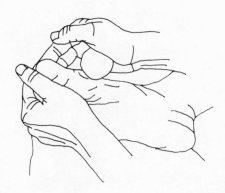

Cup the golf ball in the working hand. The fingers of the working hand are placed on top of the foot. Roll the edge of the foot with the golf ball. Make several passes.

Variation: Change the hand holding the golf ball.

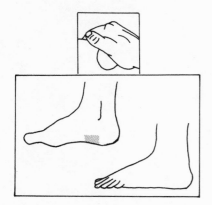
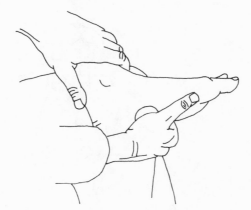

Cup the golf ball in the working hand. The fingers of the working hand rest on the outside edge of the foot. Roll the edge of the foot with the golf ball. Make several passes.

Variation: Change the hand holding the golf ball.

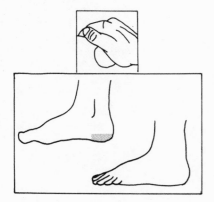
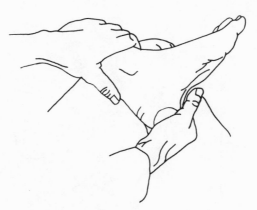

Cup the golf ball in the working hand. The fingers of the working hand rest on the outside edge of the heel. Roll the edge of the foot with the golf ball. Make several passes.

Variation: Change the hand holding the golf ball.

MISCELLANEOUS: Golf Ball

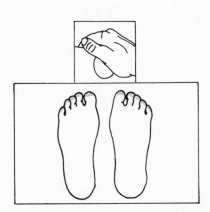

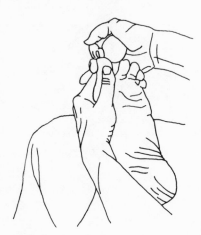

Cup the golf ball in the working hand. The big toe is trapped between the fingers of the working hand and the golf ball. Roll the big toe with the golf ball. Include the tip of the toe.

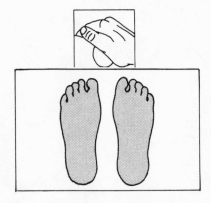

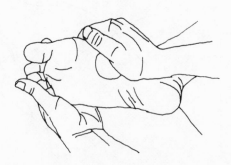

Cup the golf ball in the palm of the working hand. Steady the foot with the holding hand. Place the golf ball on the bottom of the foot and roll. Make several passes.

Variation: Change the hand holding the golf ball.

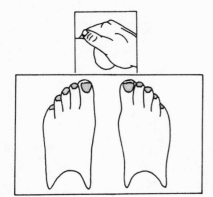

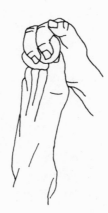

Use the same approach toward the other toes.

Cup the golf ball in the fingers of the working hand. Place the palm of the working hand on the bottom of the foot. The toes are caught between the golf ball and the palm of the hand. Roll the toe with the golf ball. Make several passes. Include rolling the ball across the nail.

MISCELLANEOUS FOOT: Foot Roller

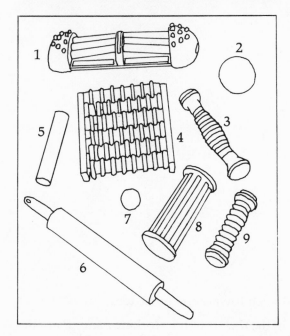

1   Step Roller®
2   Tennis Ball
3   Footsie Roller®
4   Wiehl Roller®
5   Tortilla Roller
6   Rolling Pin
7   Golf Ball
8   Case Roller®
9   Pedicure Roller

Foot rollers are available at most health food stores.

Cylindrical objects lend themselves quite well to rolling under the foot. Aside from the commercially available foot rollers, you can use objects found around the house, including a rolling pin, a soft drink bottle, or the rung of a chair. Having several cylindrical objects will allow you to station them at places where you spend time. The roller will be readily available for use. Under the dining room table or by your favorite arm chair are two convenient spots. Be careful not to put them in pathways where you walk.

Note: *Be aware of your individual response to the pressure exerted by the hard surface of a foot roller. Choose a level of pressure according to your preference and comfort level.*

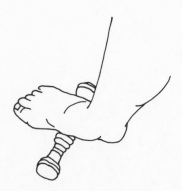
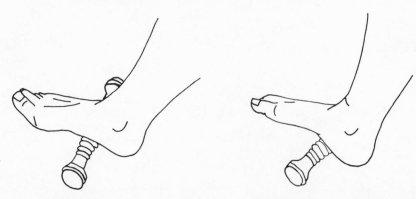

Re-positioning the foot from inside to center to outside to roll the entire foot.

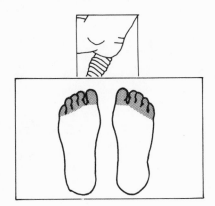

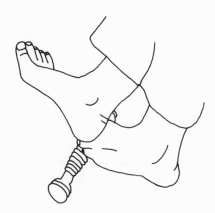

Place the heel of the opposite foot on the toe to be worked and roll. The heel provides leverage. Re-position the heel for working each toe. Experiment by turning the worked foot from side to side to work the sides of the toes.

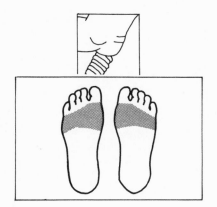

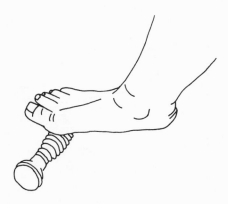

Place the foot on the roller. Roll, using a heel on top of the foot for increased pressure. Angle the foot from outside to center to inside to work the whole area.

(continued on next page)

(continued from preceding page)

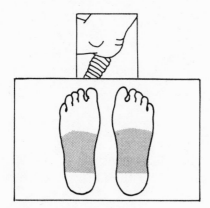

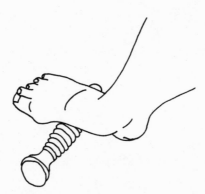

Place the foot on the roller. Roll, angling the foot from outside to center to inside. Pressure may be increased by crossing the legs.

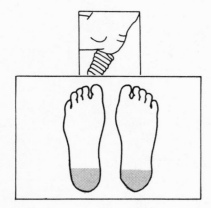

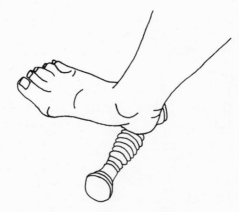

The heel is a tough area and the roller also easily slips away. For these reasons you may want to cross your legs while rolling this area to exert pressure and to control the roller. Here again, the foot may be angled to the outside, inside and center.

TECHNIQUE SUMMARY CHART: FOOT REFLEXOLOGY

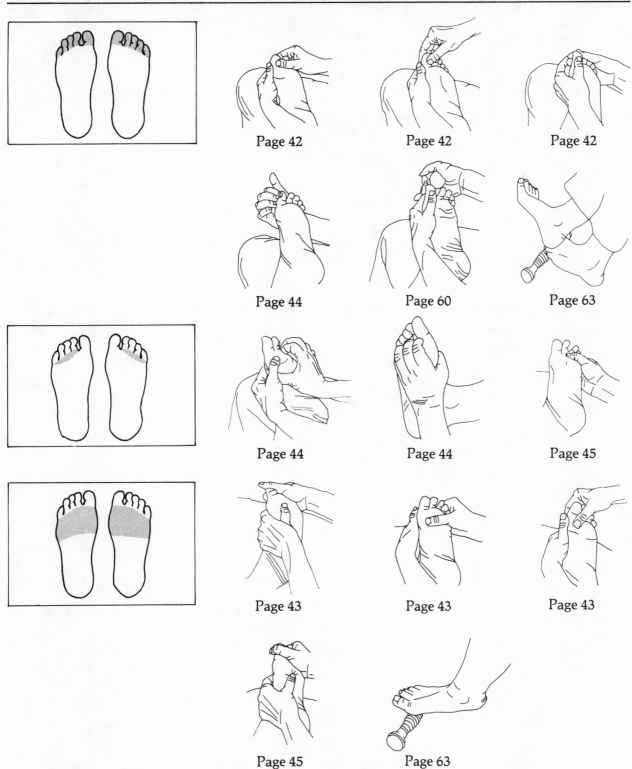

Page 42   Page 42   Page 42

Page 44   Page 60   Page 63

Page 44   Page 44   Page 45

Page 43   Page 43   Page 43

Page 45   Page 63

TECHNIQUE SUMMARY CHART: FOOT REFLEXOLOGY

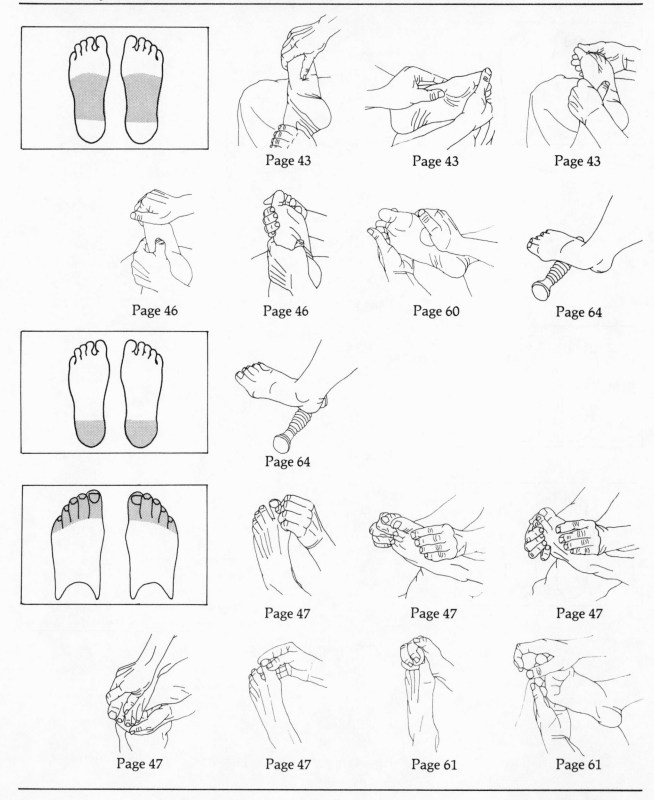

Page 43   Page 43   Page 43

Page 46   Page 46   Page 60   Page 64

Page 64

Page 47   Page 47   Page 47

Page 47   Page 47   Page 61   Page 61

TECHNIQUE SUMMARY CHART: FOOT REFLEXOLOGY

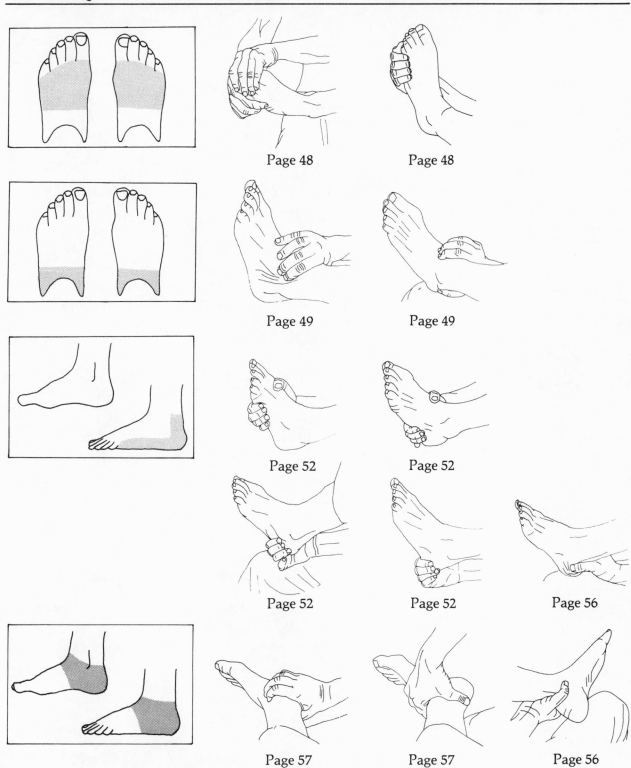

Page 48   Page 48

Page 49   Page 49

Page 52   Page 52

Page 52   Page 52   Page 56

Page 57   Page 57   Page 56

TECHNIQUE SUMMARY CHART: FOOT REFLEXOLOGY

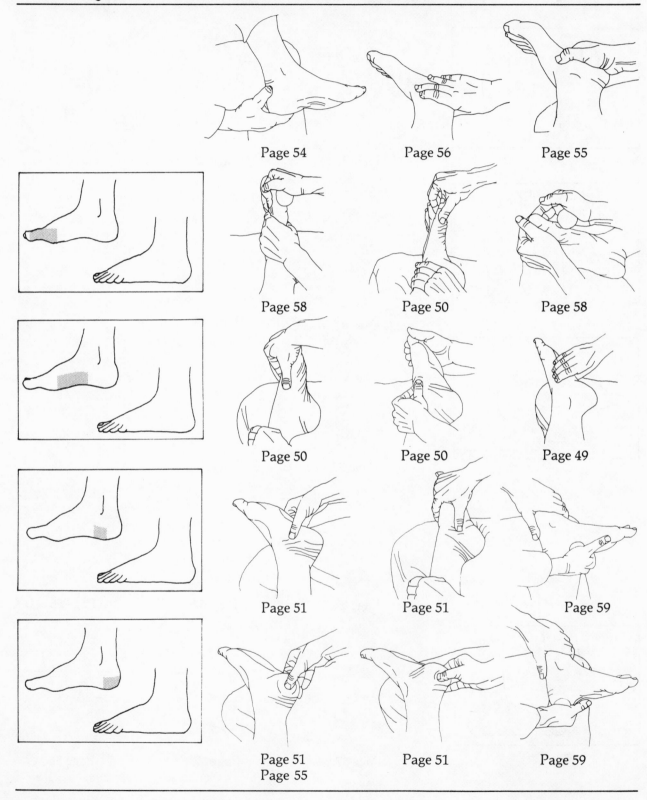

Page 54   Page 56   Page 55

Page 58   Page 50   Page 58

Page 50   Page 50   Page 49

Page 51   Page 51   Page 59

Page 51   Page 51   Page 59
Page 55

HAND REFLEXOLOGY

Applied Techniques

PALM OF HAND: Thumb Walking

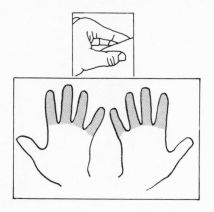

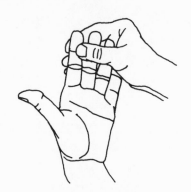

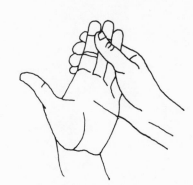

Rest the finger to be worked on the four fingers of the working hand. Use the *thumb walking* technique to make several passes. Cover the entire finger. The joints in particular are areas of interest.

Variation: Particularly effective for working around a joint.

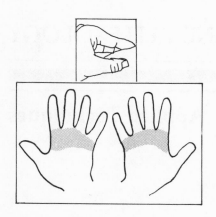

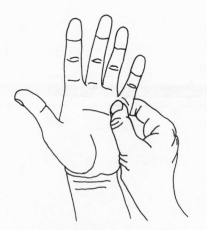

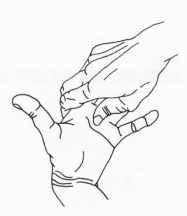

Rest the fingers of the working hand on the back of the hand to be worked. Use the *thumb walking* technique to walk up the troughs created by the metacarpal heads on the palm of the hand. Hold the fingers back on the hand being worked to better expose these troughs and to reduce the thickness or fleshiness in the area.

Variation: ↓ ←

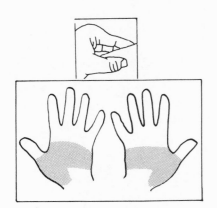

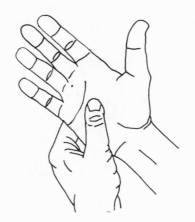

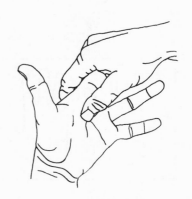

Rest the hand on the fingers of the working hand. Use the *thumb walking* technique to work through this area. Because this is a fleshy area of the hand, proper positioning of the hand being worked contributes to the ease of working. Hold the fingers back to create a firmer working surface.

Variation: ↓

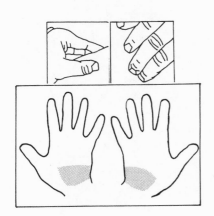

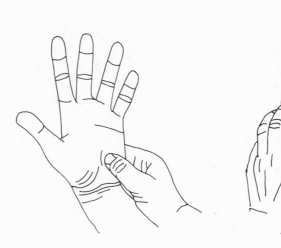

Rest the hand on the fingers of the working hand. Use the *thumb walking* technique to work through this area.

Variation: *Finger walking technique.* Grasp the wrist for leverage.

PALM OF HAND: Finger Walking/Grip Techniques

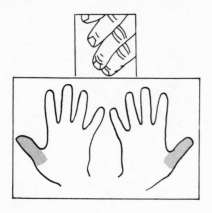

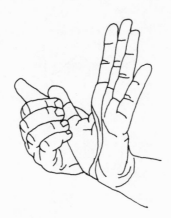

Rest the thumb to be worked in the palm of the working hand. Use the *finger walking* technique to work the area. Make successive passes to cover the palm surface of the thumb.

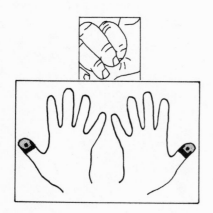

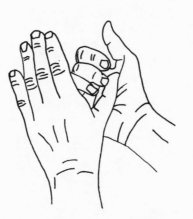

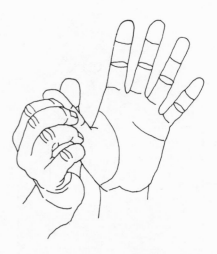

Place the thumb to be worked in the palm of the working hand. Place the tip of the index or middle finger on the area to be worked. Using the *single finger grip* technique, exert an alternating pressure on the area. Be aware of finger nails. Re-position the working finger and repeat.

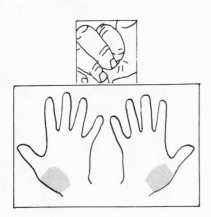

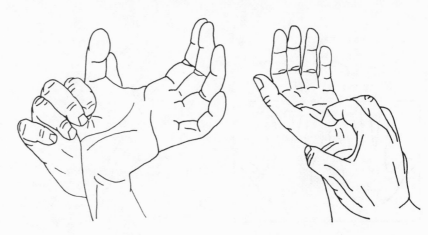

Rest the hand to be worked on the palm of the working hand. Place the tip of the index finger on the area to be worked. Use the *single finger grip* technique to exert an alternating pressure. Be aware of fingernails. Re-position the working finger and repeat.

Variation: Grasp the hand to be worked at the wrist.

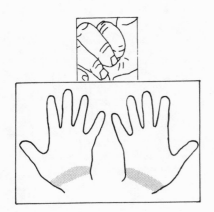

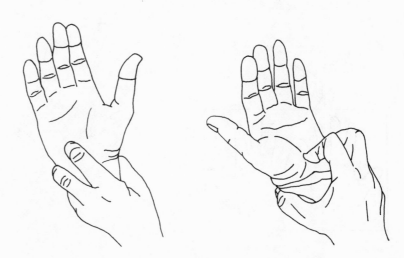

Grasp the wrist. Place the tip of the index finger on the area to be worked. Use the *single finger grip* technique to create an alternating pressure. Be aware of fingernails. Re-position the working finger and repeat.

PALM OF HAND: Multiple Finger Grip

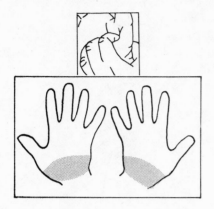

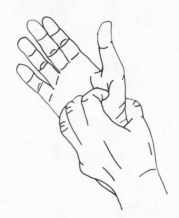

Place the heel of the working hand on the top of the hand, below the thumb, providing leverage for the working fingers. Place the finger tips on the palm of the hand. Use the *multiple finger grip* technique to work the fleshy part of the hand. Be aware of nails. Re-position the working fingers and repeat.

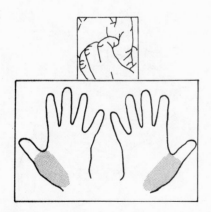

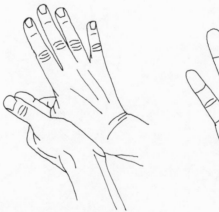

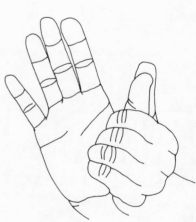

Place the heel of the working hand on the wrist. Wrap the thumb around the wrist for leverage. Place the finger tips on the palm of the hand. Use the *multiple finger grip* technique to work the heel of the hand. Be aware of nails. Re-position the working fingers and repeat.

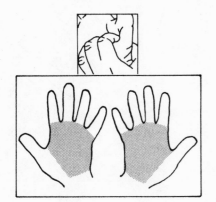

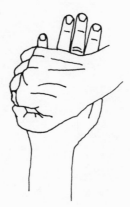

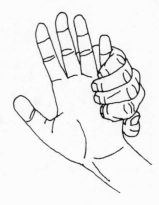

Place the heel of the working hand on top of the hand below the little finger. Place the tips of the fingers on the palm of the hand being worked. Use the *multiple finger grip* technique to work the area. Be aware of nails. Re-position the working fingers and repeat.

PALM OF HAND: Grip Techniques

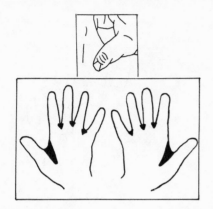

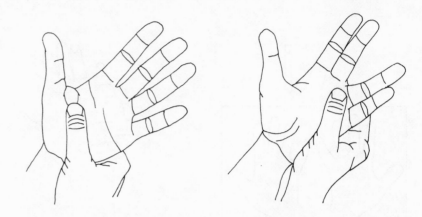

Grasp the hand, positioning the thumb and finger in opposition to each other as if to pinch the webbing of the hand. Use the *thumb walking* technique to work through the area. Make successive passes. Be aware of nails.

Variation: Use the *pinch grip* technique.

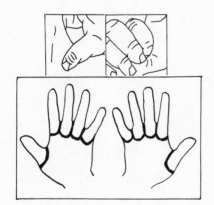

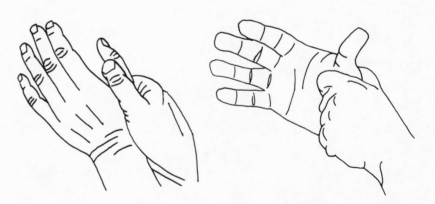

Grasp the hand to be worked with the thumb and index finger of the working hand. The second joint of the index finger is the point of contact. Use the thumb for support and leverage and the joint of the index finger as the working joint. Place the index finger under the joint below the thumb. Rotate the working hand back and forth, digging into the joint with the index finger.

Variation: Use the *single finger grip* technique.

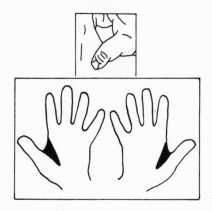

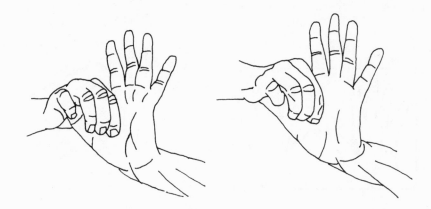

Place the thumb and finger on the webbing of the hand. To use the *pinch grip* technique, exert pressure by pinching the thumb and finger together. The tip of the finger exerts a greater pressure than the thumb tip which is used more as a backstop.

Variation: *Finger walking* technique.

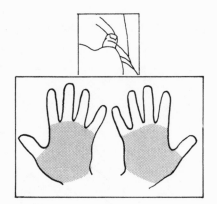

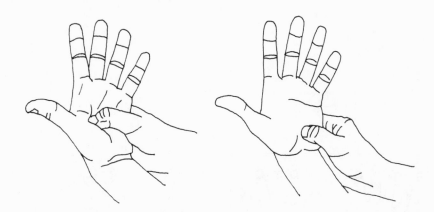

Grasp the hand, positioning the thumb on the palm of the hand and fingers on top of the hand in opposition to each other (as if to pinch the hand). To use the *pinch grip* technique, try to pinch the thumb and fingers together, pumping to create alternating pressure. The thumb exerts a greater pressure than the fingers. Be aware of nails.

Variation: *Thumb walking* technique.

TOP OF HAND: Pinch Grip

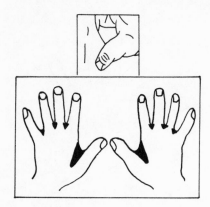

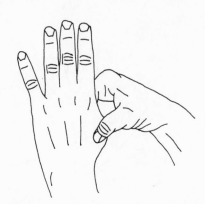

Place the thumb and finger on the webbing of the hand. To use the *pinch grip* technique, exert pressure by pinching the thumb and finger together. Be aware of fingernails. The tip of the thumb exerts a greater pressure than the finger tip which is used more as a backstop.

Variation: Create alternating deep pressure by pumping with the thumb and finger.

Variation: *Thumb walking* technique.

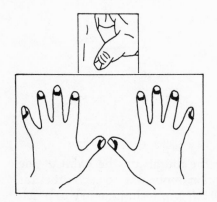

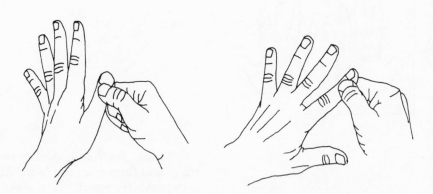

Position the thumb to be worked between the index finger (second joint) and thumb. To use the *pinch grip* technique, exert pressure by pinching the thumb and finger together.

TOP OF HAND: Thumb Walking

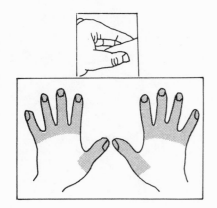

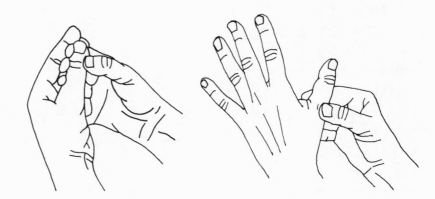

The *thumb walking* technique is used to work the fingers and thumb of the opposite hand. The fingers of the working hand provide support and leverage. To begin, rest the thumb of the hand to be worked on the four fingers of the working thumb hand. Using the *thumb walking* technique, make several passes to cover the entire thumb, including the nail and the sides. The joints in particular are areas for exploration. Change hands and work the other thumb in a similar manner. Return to the original hand and follow the above procedure to work the index finger.

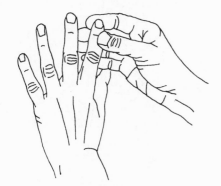

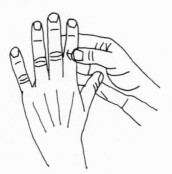

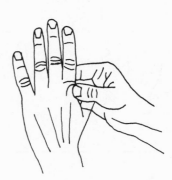

Alternate between the two hands covering the topside of each digit. A pattern of alternation is followed to make the work less tiring for the working thumb.

TOP OF HAND: Miscellaneous

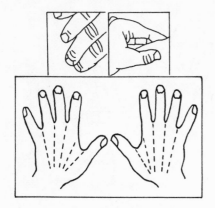

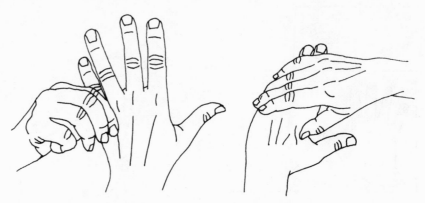

Place the thumb of the working hand in the palm of the other hand. Use the *finger walking* technique to walk down each side of the trough between two metacarpal bones on top of the hand. Begin at the base of the finger and work from the joint at the base of the finger into the wrist. Work both the side of the trough to the outside of the hand and the side of the trough to the inside. Work each trough in a similar manner. The trough between the thumb and index finger is wider than the others. Use the *finger walking* technique to make several passes through this area, both on the index finger side and the thumb side of the trough.

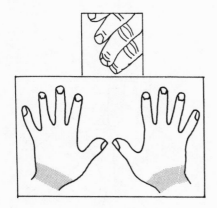

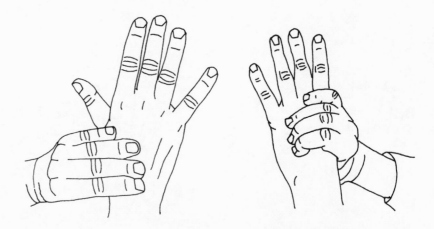

Rest the hand to be worked on the thumb of the working hand. Use the *finger walking* technique to walk across the hand. Make several passes. Include the wrist.

Variation: *Multiple finger walking* technique.

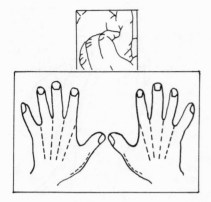
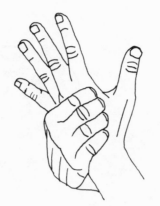
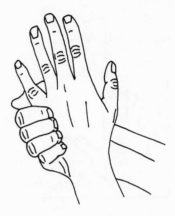

Place the heel of the working hand on the palm of the hand below the little finger. This provides the leverage for this technique. Position the tips of the fingers in the trough between the little finger and its neighbor. Rotate the wrist of the hand being worked to allow the working fingers to work the trough. Work the other troughs in a similar manner.

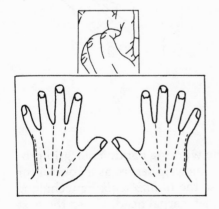
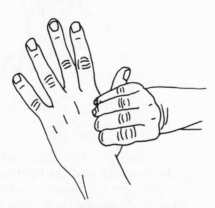

To work the other side of the troughs, re-position the working hand so that the heel of the hand is on the palm below the thumb. Work as above.

SIDES OF HAND: Thumb Walking/Finger Walking

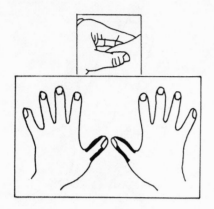

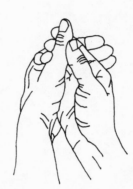

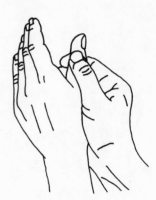

Rest the thumb to be worked on the fingers of the working hand. Use the *thumb walking* technique to walk up the thumb. Reposition the working thumb and make several passes.

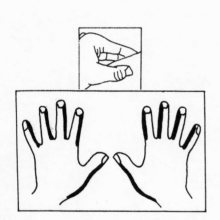

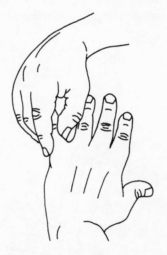

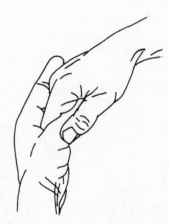

Grasp the little finger with the working hand. Your grip provides leverage and the tightness of the grip serves as a control for the pressure you wish to exert. Use the *thumb walking* technique to walk down the finger into the metacarpal head. Grasp the next finger and work the same way. The thumb must be free to walk while you maintain your grasp with the fingers and the rest of the hand, thereby providing leverage. Work the other fingers in a similar manner.

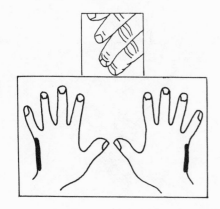 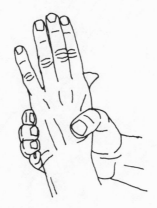 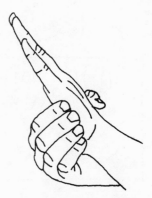

Grasp the hand to be worked. The thumb of the **working** hand provides leverage. Use the *multiple finger walking* **technique** to walk through the area.

Variation: *Single finger walking* technique. *Rotating on a point* technique.

MISCELLANEOUS HAND: Rotating on a Point

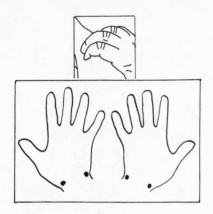

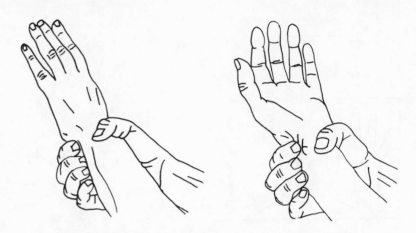

With the palm of the hand to be worked turned down, grasp the wrist with the thumb on the palm side. To use the *rotating on a point* technique, locate the point with the index finger and rotate the wrist several times, first in a clockwise direction and then a counter-clockwise direction. With the palm of the hand to be worked turned up, grasp the wrist with the thumb on the palm side and repeat.

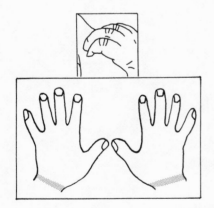

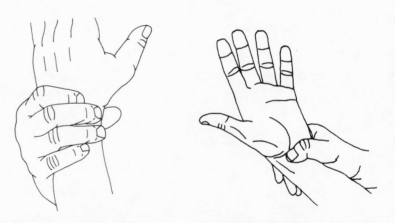

With the hand to be worked palm down, grasp the wrist with the thumb on the palm side and the fingers on the top side. To use the *rotating on a point* technique, the index finger pinpoints an area and remains stationary as the wrist of the hand being worked is rotated several times in both directions. This should create an on/off pressure with the index finger. The thumb and the working hand provide the leverage.

Variation: *Rotating on a point* technique with the thumb.

MISCELLANEOUS HAND: Buffing

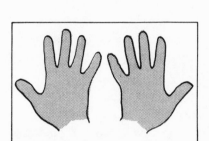
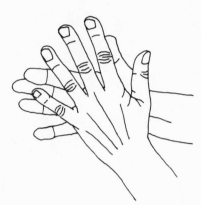
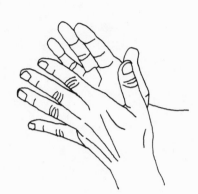

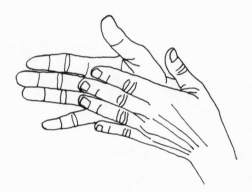
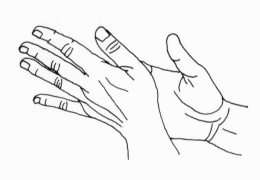

The object of buffing is to move one hand across the other in a rapid, repetitive manner. Buffing is a general technique of use for circulation and general stimulation.

(continued on next page)

(continued from preceding page)

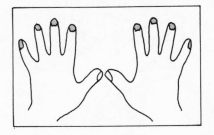

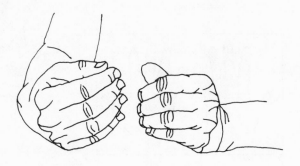

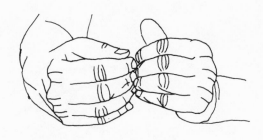

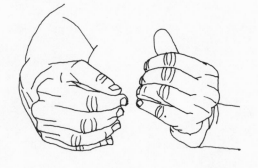

Nail buffing — The fingernails of one hand are moved rapidly and repetitively across the nails of the other hand.

MISCELLANEOUS HAND: Golf Ball

A golf ball is used for working the hands because it's of appropriate size and both inexpensive and easy to use. In general, round or cylindrical objects work well because they roll smoothly over the surface. Choose an object that works well for you. But *remember* that you are *never* to use an object such as a golf ball on someone else! Be aware of your individual response to the pressure exerted by the hard surface of the golf ball. Choose a level of pressure according to your preference and comfort level.

To be effective using a golf ball on the hands, one must learn to control it in order to create a stable working surface. This is achieved by cupping the ball in the working hand or wedging it between the two hands. Another element, not only adding to control of the ball but also providing leverage and control of pressure exerted, is the placement of the four fingers on top of the hand. The golf ball is thus trapped between the palmar surfaces of the two hands, with control of pressure by the fingers.

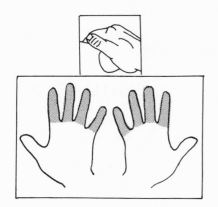

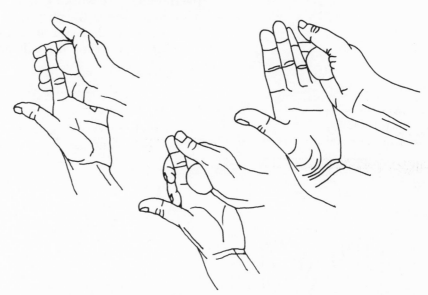

Cup the golf ball in the working hand. The finger to be worked is trapped between the golf ball and the fingers of the working hand. Roll the finger with the golf ball. Make succeeding passes until the length of the finger has been covered. Leverage and pressure are varied by tightening the grasp of the working hand.

Go to the next finger. Cup the finger to be worked in the working hand and proceed as above. Continue through the other fingers.

(continued on next page)

(continued from preceding page)

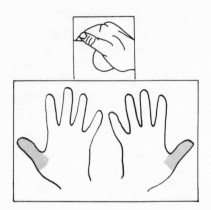

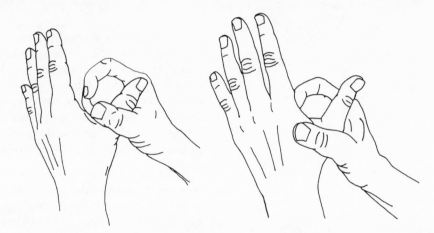

The thumb presents a different situation for the working hand. Hold the golf ball with the first two fingers of the working hand. Place the golf ball on the palmar surface of the thumb. Place the thumb of the working hand on top of the thumb to be worked. This thumb serves the purpose of creating leverage and controlling pressure. Now that you have a stable working surface, move the working hand to roll the ball across the thumb.

Cover the length of the thumb with succeeding passes. Include the tip of the thumb, the ball, the joints and the shaft of the thumb.

Variation: Work as above but move the hand being worked to roll the ball across the thumb.

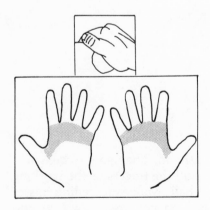

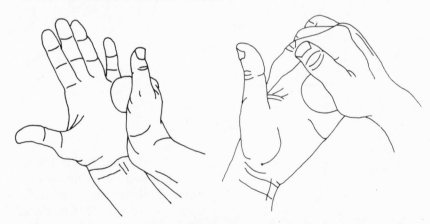

Cup the golf ball in the working hand. Place the fingers of the working hand on top of the hand to be worked. Roll the golf ball around and into the trough created by the heads of the metacarpal bones. Work the two troughs to the outside of the hand in this manner.

The two troughs to the inside of the hand are difficult to work in a similar manner because of the lessened ability to exert pressure and provide leverage with the extended reach. To counter this, reposition the working hand to the inside of the hand being worked on. Cup the golf ball in the working hand with the fingers placed on top of the hand being worked. Roll the ball around and through the two troughs.

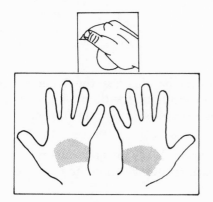

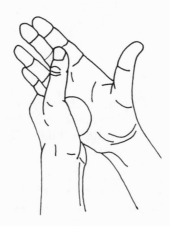

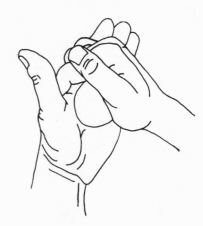

Cup the golf ball in the working hand. Roll the ball. Tighten or loosen the grasp of the working hand to vary pressure.

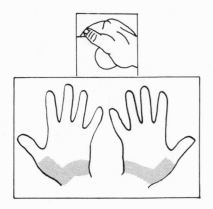

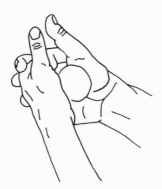

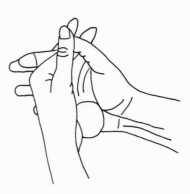

Interlace the fingers of the two hands as if praying. Place the golf ball so that it is held between the heels of the two hands. Roll the ball. Tighten or loosen the grasp of the hands to vary pressure.

(continued on next page)

(continued from preceding page)

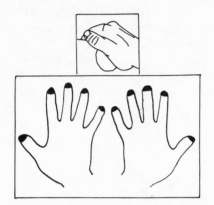

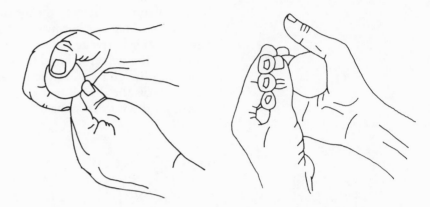

Cup the golf ball in the palm of the hand. Wrap the fingers of the working hand around the thumb, trapping the thumb between the fingers and golf ball. Tighten or loosen the grip of the fingers to vary pressure.

Grasp the golf ball with two fingers. Place the golf ball on the fingernail. Roll the golf ball from side to side varying the pressure with the grip of the fingers.

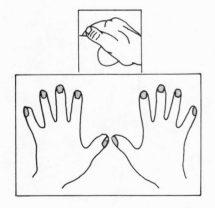

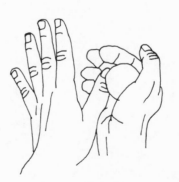

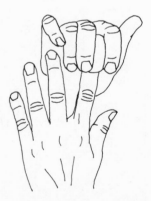

Cup the golf ball in the hand. Wrap the fingers of the working hand around the thumb, trapping the thumb between the fingers and golf ball. Tighten or loosen the grip of the fingers to vary pressure.

TECHNIQUE SUMMARY CHART: HAND REFLEXOLOGY

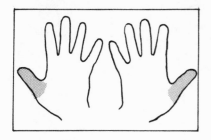

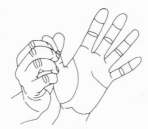

Page 72

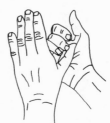

Page 72

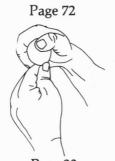

Page 90

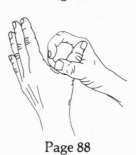

Page 88

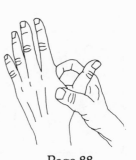

Page 88

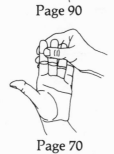

Page 70

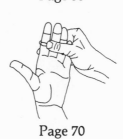

Page 70

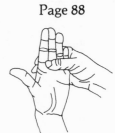

Page 70

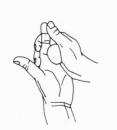

Page 87

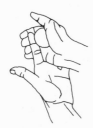

Page 87

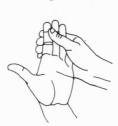

Page 70

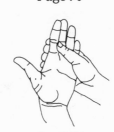

Page 70

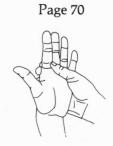

Page 70

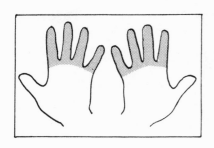

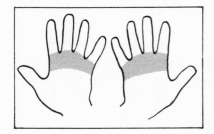

Page 70

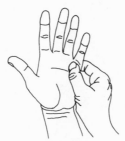

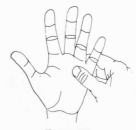

Page 70

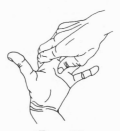

Page 70

TECHNIQUE SUMMARY CHART: HAND REFLEXOLOGY

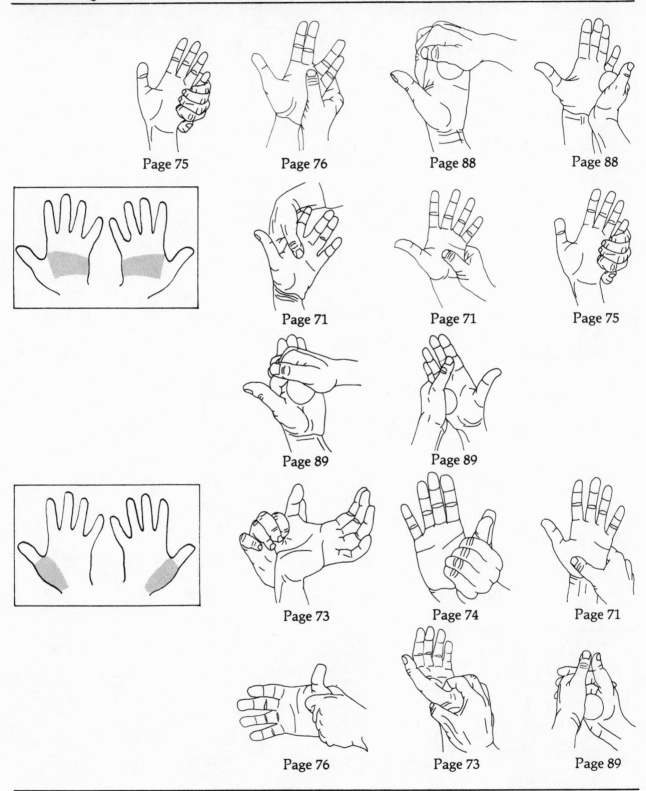

Page 75

Page 76

Page 88

Page 88

Page 71

Page 71

Page 75

Page 89

Page 89

Page 73

Page 74

Page 71

Page 76

Page 73

Page 89

TECHNIQUE SUMMARY CHART: HAND REFLEXOLOGY

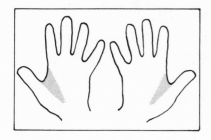

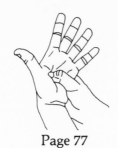

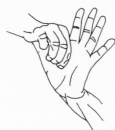

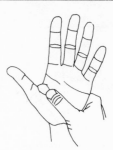

Page 77

Page 77

Page 76

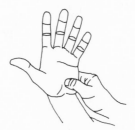

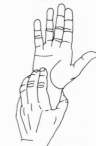

Page 71

Page 71

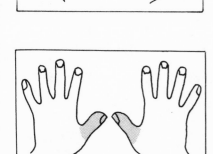

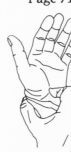

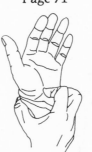

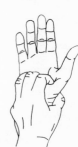

Page 73

Page 73

Page 74

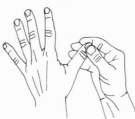

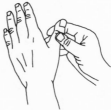

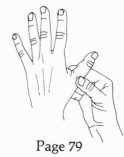

Page 79

Page 79

Page 79

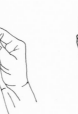

Page 78

Page 90

TECHNIQUE SUMMARY CHART: HAND REFLEXOLOGY

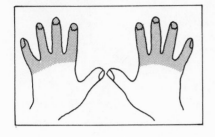

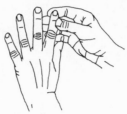

Page 79

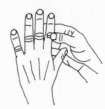

Page 79

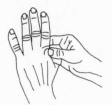

Page 79

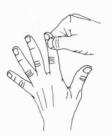

Page 78

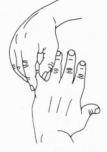

Page 83

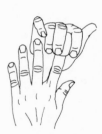

Page 90

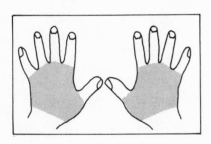

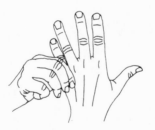

Page 80

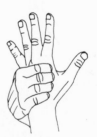

Page 81

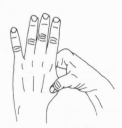

Page 78

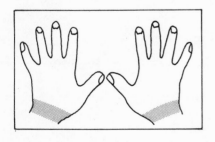

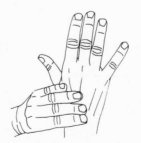

Page 80

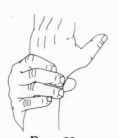

Page 82

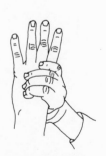

Page 80

Stride Replication

INTRODUCTION

The validity of reflexology has always been founded in providing the sensory experiences of light touch, deep pressure, angulation of joints, muscle and tendon stretch, and the rate of stretch. These are all, with the exception of light touch, forms of communication necessary for movement. To further encourage variety in this communication, we have developed a set of techniques which we refer to as *stride replication*. As this phrase implies, the techniques mimic some of the key sensory signals necessary for walking or standing.

Stride replication techniques are a recognition of two important elements of walking: (1) directional movement of the foot, and (2) weight bearing. The foot's role in walking is to shift direction while signaling the body to shift weight in response. *Stride replication* mimicks key sensory signals necessary for walking. Through *stride replication* techniques, these key signals are exaggerated. The extremes of basic directional movements are practiced and the foot relaxes in response.

As with any sensory organ, the foot receives information through sensory experience. The eye, for example, is a sensory organ which processes light as bits of information necessary for vision. The foot as a sensory organ processes stretch and pressure as bits of information necessary for locomotion. When driving, the sight of a stop sign evokes an all but unconscious response of reaching for the brake pedal with the foot. This is an integration of the eye seeing the stop sign and the foot making a proper response. A movement is made possible by organized packets of information from the sensory organs. The foot, too, gathers packets of information which are necessary for an integrated activity. Here the activity is standing or walking. This is no trivial task. It can be accomplished with ease only by the contraction and relaxation of specific muscle groups throughout the body. To make locomotion possible, these muscle groups respond in sequence. The sequences are signalled by a particular sensory event: the pressure of the surface being walked on, the perceived angle of the terrain, the stretch of the muscle in response to the surface, and the speed at which the surface is encountered. The sensory signal and the resulting action of muscle groups is referred to as one phase of the stride mechanism. Adaptation to shoes and modern surfaces has forced the stride mechanism to be performed within limited patterns.

The beginning of one such phase is the heel strike. When the heel strikes the floor, it communicates information to the entire body about the position of the foot in relationship to the body. It signals a moment in the stride mechanism where it is necessary for the foot to accept the body's weight. Each foot step requires this information.

DESCRIPTION OF A FOOT STEP:

Heel strike: the foots first contact with surface at heel strike. The foot is in a flexible position for the purpose of perceiving what is underfoot. Specifically, at the point of heel strike, the decision must be made of the angle at which the foot should meet the terrain. Adjustments can thus be made to make possible, for example, walking across sand versus hiking uphill.

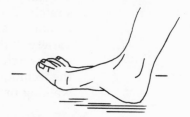

heel on ground

Stance phase: the shifting of the body weight from the heel to the ball of the foot. The stance phase is so-named to note that, at this point of the footstep, the body stands on one foot, accepting its total weight.

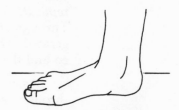

foot flat on ground

Toe-off: the final thrust by the toes as the foot leaves the ground. In this final phase of a foot step, the ball of the foot and toes lever the body weight off the ground.

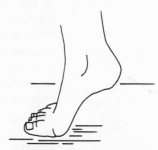

ball of foot on ground

"A footstep is a stumble caught in time."
Sir Charles Sherrington

Direction and weight bearing are important elements of a foot step. The four directional movements in a foot step are dorsiflexion, inversion, eversion and plantarflexion. In a normal foot step, the foot moves through all four directions. Movements such as pointing the toe, rotating the ankle or moving the foot from side to side are not required in our everyday activities.

The restrictive environment of shoe wear and flat surfaces causes the muscle groups involved in locomotion to move within limited ranges of motion. The net result is a loss of practice in the fine-tuning capabilities of the foot.

ACCENTUATING THE DIRECTIONAL MOVEMENTS OF THE FOOT

These exercises move the foot through the directional phases of a foot step.

Guided direction

D O R S I F L E X I O N

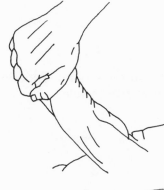

Sit with one foot crossed over the opposite leg. Use the opposite hand (left hand for right foot and vice versa) to grasp the ball of the foot and toes. Use the heel of the hand to bend the toes and the entire foot back.

E V E R S I O N

Wrap the hand around the foot. When turning the foot, the heel of the hand exerts an upward pressure as the fingers pull in a downward direction. The bottom of the foot should now more fully be turned towards you.

P L A N T A R F L E X I O N

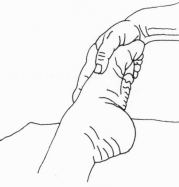

Sit with one leg crossed over the other. grasp the ball and toes of the foot. The fingers rest on the top of the foot as the heel of the hand pushes down on the foot and points the toes.

I N V E R S I O N

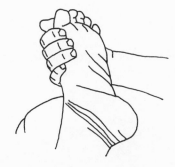

Wrap the hand around the foot. The fingers wrap around the little toe side of the foot. Pull the outside edge of the foot up with the fingers as you push in a downward direction with the heel of the hand. A maximum effect can be achieved by pushing on the joint of the foot at the base of the big toe.

(continued on next page)

ACCENTUATING THE DIRECTIONAL MOVEMENTS OF THE FOOT

(continued from preceding page)

Working against a surface

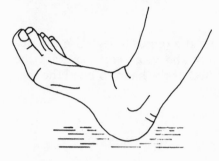

While seated, place the heel on the ground. Pull back on the toes. Using the heel as a pivot point, experiment and rock the foot back and forth, side to side.

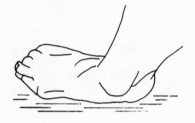

Place the inside edge of the foot on the ground. Experiment and rock the foot back and forth, from side to side.

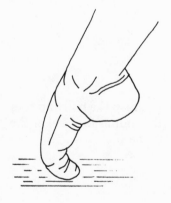

Place the tops of the toes on the ground. Experiment and rock the foot back and forth, from side to side.

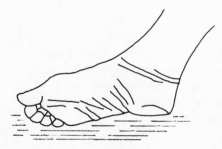

Place the outside edge of the foot on the ground. Experiment and rock the foot back and forth, from side to side.

Practicing rotation

DORSIFLEXION

Draw a circle in the air with big toe. Circle the foot in both directions, first one and then the other. Was it difficult to turn the ankle? In which direction was it easier to move? Was the circle a complete one? Are parts of the circle more difficult than others?

EVERSION

Think of the circle drawn by the big toe as a clock face with the 12, the 3, the 6 and the 9 the four basic directional movements of the foot. With the big toe in the 12 o'clock position, the foot is in dorsiflexion. The right foot is in eversion at the 3 o'clock position, plantarflexion at 6 o'clock and inversion at the 9 o'clock.

Draw a circle in the air with the big toe. Note which portion of the circle was the tightest. Was it the 12 o'clock to 3 o'clock portion? The 3 to 6 o'clock? the 6 to 9 'clock? The 9 to 12 o'clock?

On the left foot, the foot is in dorsiflexion at 12 o'clock position, inversion at the 3 o'clock, plantarflexion at the 6 o'clock and eversion at the 9 o'clock.

PLANTARFLEXION

INVERSION

To practice movement in, for example, the 12 to 3 o'clock portion of the circle, grasp the foot as shown in the dorsiflexion illustration. Draw a circle in the air. The big toe etches the circle while the hand moves the foot.

Other portions of the circle may be practiced in a similar manner by changing the position of the guiding hand as shown in the other directional illustrations.

VARIETY OF SENSORY SIGNALS

The techniques of cupping, tapping and percussion are applied to the feet to provide a variety of sensory signals. The foot is placed in one of the four directional positions to enhance the variety.

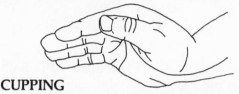

CUPPING

In cupping, the hand pockets air to form a muffled clap. To begin, cup your hand as though scooping water from a stream. To practice the technique, clap the cupped hands together. The sound made should be a dull thud.

Try this technique on the foot. The cup of the hand should be shaped to the foot surface for maximum effect. This is achieved by varying the curve of the fingers. If the sound of the technique is more of a slap and the foot is made red, the hand is too open and the fingers not curved enough. Apply the technique to the areas indicated (see chart). The ankle is a key area for application.

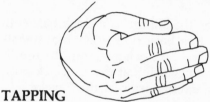

TAPPING

In the technique of tapping, the outside of the little finger of an open, relaxed hand makes contact with the foot. The effect is like rapping a closed hand-fan on the knee. The ribs of the fan rap together. In tapping, the fingers of the hand tap together. To achieve this effect, the fingers must be relaxed (rather than stiff as in a karate chop).

To practice tapping, try this technique on your thigh. Keep the hand open and the fingers relaxed. Can you hear the fingers slap together making a "tap, tap, tapping" sound? The goal of tapping is achieved by a rapid, rhythmic stroke rather than a forceful blow. Force may cause injury or discomfort.

The movement of the working arm is the same as that used in the technique of percussion. The bicep of the arm is flexed and the arm is turned so that the outside of the hand may make contact with the foot. Unlike percussion, the hand is open and the contact is made with the outside of the little finger. The elbow is the only moving part of the working arm. The bicep remains flexed throughout.

Apply the technique to the areas indicated on the foot.

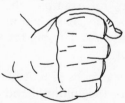

PERCUSSION

Form the hand into a loose fist. The object of the technique is to make contact with the padded, outside edge of the hand on targeted areas on the foot. (See chart) The elbow is the only moving part of the working arm. The bicep remains flexed throughout. Draw the right arm towards the chest and swing it forward, making contact with the area on the foot. Set up a rhythm. Don't try to use too much force. Force is not as important as a rapid stretch of the muscle. The tempo, which can be established by the flexing of the bicep throughout the technique, is of more importance than force.

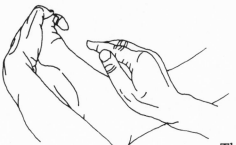
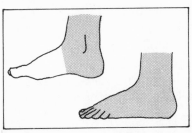
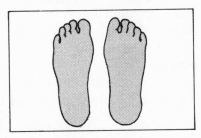

The technique of *cupping* is directed at the ankle. The ankle reports important information on its position. The reporters are the proprioceptors which sense joint angulation and muscle and tendon stretch. The ability of these reporters is not fully utilized if there is no "news", if certain movements are never made. Without practice, the fine movements become more and more difficult to perform.

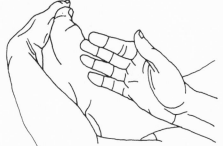
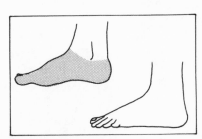
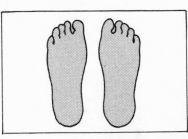

In the technique of *tapping*, the foot is held back in the stretched position. The application of tapping replicates the important moment in walking. The message is one of extreme stretch. The application of rapid tapping signals to the brain that an extreme stretch is occuring. In an effort to accommodate this motion, the brain signals the muscle groups involved to widen the range of motion. In essence, *tapping* is an attempt to break the pattern of set demands routinely experienced in flat surface walking.

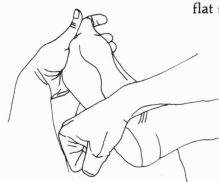
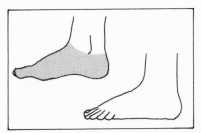
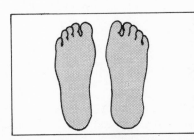

Percussion is the replication of the sensory information received by the foot as the heel and other parts of the foot strike the surface. Just as in the actual stride mechanism, the sensory input triggers a response from the entire body. The ultimate response is one of relaxation.

VARIETY OF SENSORY SIGNAL/Directional movement of the foot

Use the holding hand to place the foot in one of the four basic directional positions. Choose one of the three sensory signals and with the working hand, apply it.

Use the chart to explore the possibilities of direction and sensory signal.

Variation: With the working hand, grasp a tennis ball. Tap gently on the foot with the ball to create a sensory signal.

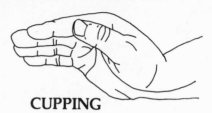

CUPPING

DIRECTIONAL MOVEMENTS

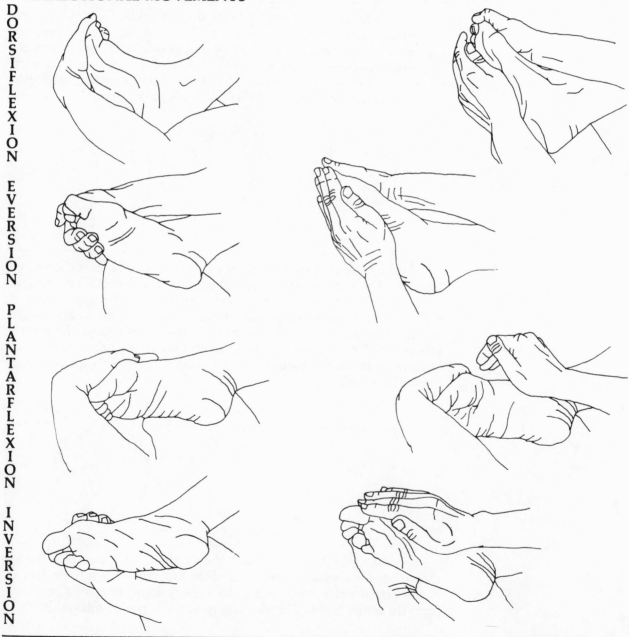

DORSIFLEXION   EVERSION   PLANTARFLEXION   INVERSION

TAPPING PERCUSSION

DORSIFLEXION EVERSION PLANTARFLEXION INVERSION

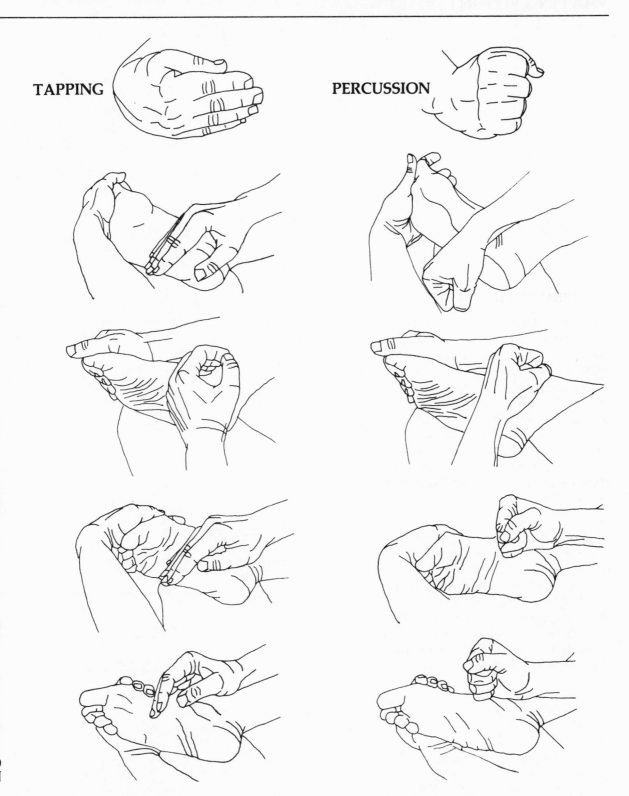

VARYING WEIGHT BEARING

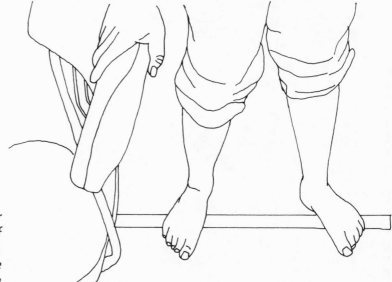

WALKING STICK

This technique is not for everyone. It creates a great deal of challenge for the foot and is, therefore, not recommended for those who have foot problems or find it an excessively painful technique. The object of the technique is to create a challenging new terrain for the foot. Use a dowel stick or broom stick to create the effect and challenge the muscles and ligaments on the bottom of the foot.

To practice, begin with a dowel stick of a smaller size (1/4″ diameter). To support yourself, grasp a stationary object such as a chair. A rug or towel laid over the stick provides padding if needed. Gently walk on the stick, feeling the effect from heel to toe. Stand in place, sensing the pressure to various parts of the foot. Walk in place, feeling the pressure.

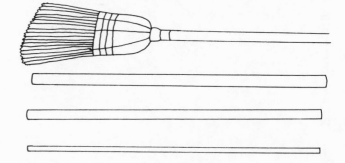

Try a variety of walking patterns such as; walking pigeon-toed, and walking with the toes pointing outward. Also, walk along the length of the stick. **Never attempt this without support.**

Two interesting areas are at the beginning of the heel and across the metatarsal arch. The sensory signal of deep pressure applied to the bottom of the foot has an effect on the entire body. Deep pressure signals that an adjustment of body position is needed. When walking across a rocky terrain, for example, continuous adjustments are made in response to what is underfoot. The response is made according to the location of pressure on the bottom of the foot.

Walking across sand may be the most familiar example of terrain underfoot affecting the rest of the body. Hiking uphill is another example of foot position accommodating the terrain, with ramifications for the entire body.

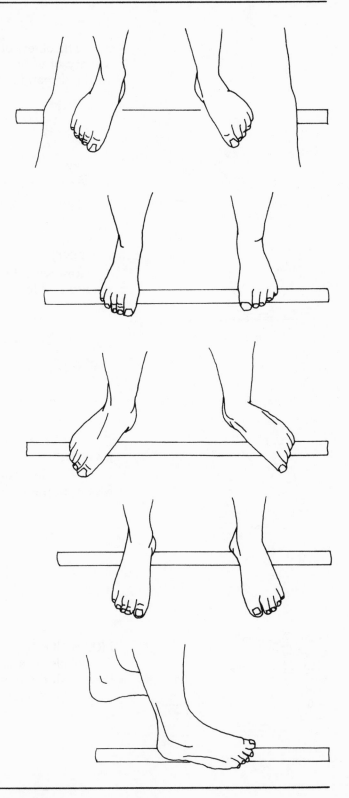

VARYING WEIGHT BEARING

The object of these weight bearing techniques is to practice a variety of weight bearing situations, from simply standing at rest to the demands of walking with a varied terrain.

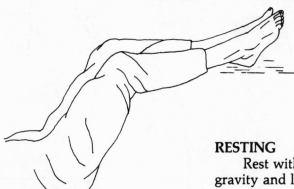

RESTING
Rest with the legs elevated to compensate for the demands of gravity and long periods of standing or walking.

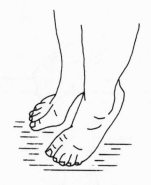

RAISING
While in a standing position, grasp a chair to ensure balance. Rise onto the balls of the foot.

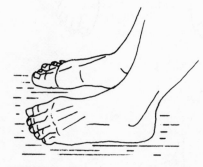

PRESSING
While in a standing or seated position, press down on the floor with the toes.

ACCENTUATING DIRECTIONAL MOVEMENT OF THE HAND

The object of the technique is to practice basic directional movements of the hand. These directions are similar to those discussed with the feet.

A series of directional movements may be practiced in a manner similar to the series with the feet.

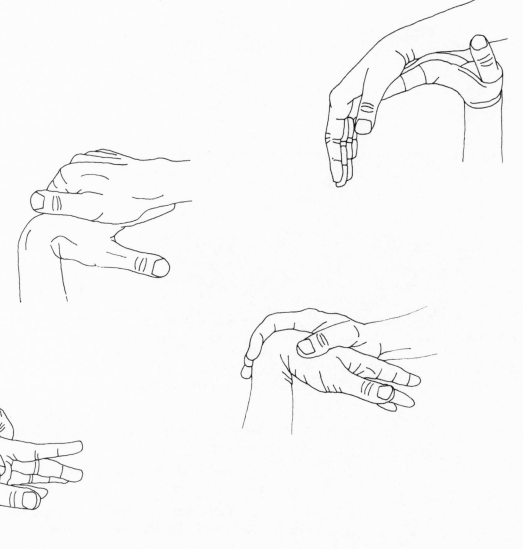

VARIETY OF SENSORY SIGNAL

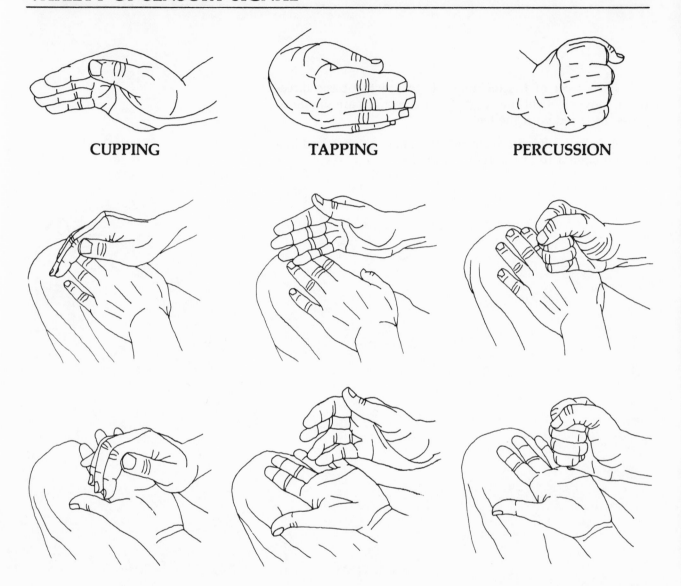

CUPPING   **TAPPING**   **PERCUSSION**

Rest the hand on the leg with the palm up or down. Select one of the three sensory signals and, with the working hand, apply it.

Use the chart to explore sensory signals as applied to the palm or top of the hand.

Variation: Hold the hand in the air. With the working hand, apply the tapping technique.

Variation: With the working hand, grasp a tennis ball. Tap gently on the hand.

CHARTS

Glossary of Symbols
Technique Pattern Charts

FOOT REFLEXOLOGY CHARTS

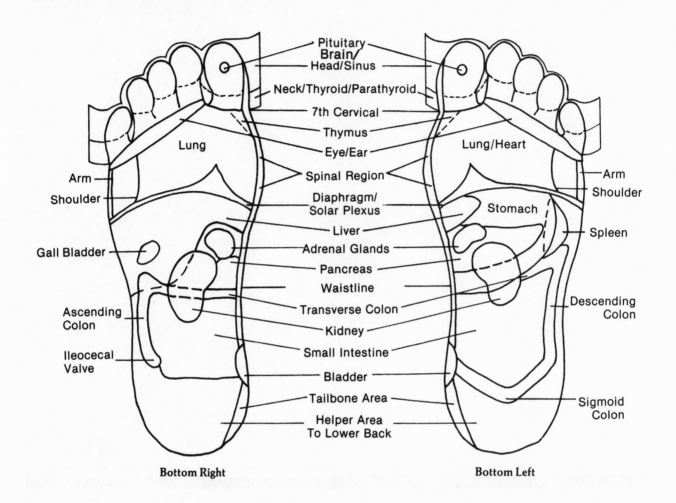

Pituitary
Brain/
Head/Sinus
Neck/Thyroid/Parathyroid
7th Cervical
Thymus
Lung
Eye/Ear
Lung/Heart
Arm
Spinal Region
Arm
Shoulder
Diaphragm/
Shoulder
Solar Plexus
Stomach
Liver
Spleen
Adrenal Glands
Gall Bladder
Pancreas
Waistline
Ascending
Transverse Colon
Descending
Colon
Kidney
Colon
Ileocecal
Small Intestine
Valve
Bladder
Tailbone Area
Sigmoid
Helper Area
Colon
To Lower Back

Bottom Right　　　　　　　　　　　　**Bottom Left**

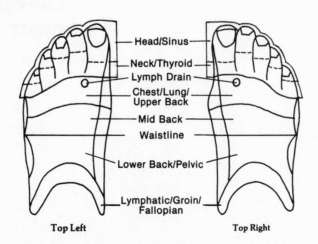

Head/Sinus
Neck/Thyroid
Lymph Drain
Chest/Lung/
Upper Back
Mid Back
Waistline
Lower Back/Pelvic
Lymphatic/Groin/
Fallopian

Top Left　　　　　　　　**Top Right**

HAND REFLEXOLOGY CHARTS

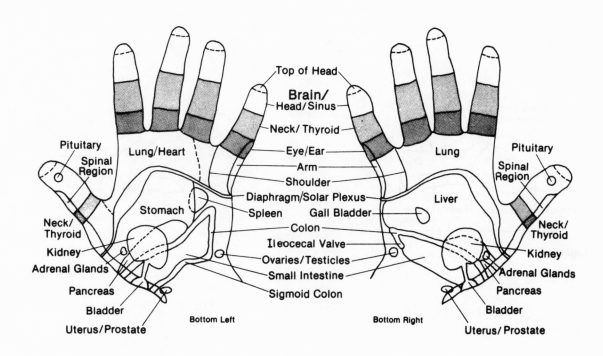

Top of Head

Brain/
Head/Sinus

Neck/Thyroid

Eye/Ear

Arm

Shoulder

Diaphragm/Solar Plexus

Spleen — Gall Bladder

Colon

Ileocecal Valve

Ovaries/Testicles

Small Intestine

Sigmoid Colon

Pituitary

Spinal Region

Lung/Heart

Neck/Thyroid

Kidney

Adrenal Glands

Pancreas

Bladder

Uterus/Prostate

Stomach

Bottom Left

Lung

Liver

Pituitary

Spinal Region

Neck/Thyroid

Kidney

Adrenal Glands

Pancreas

Bladder

Uterus/Prostate

Bottom Right

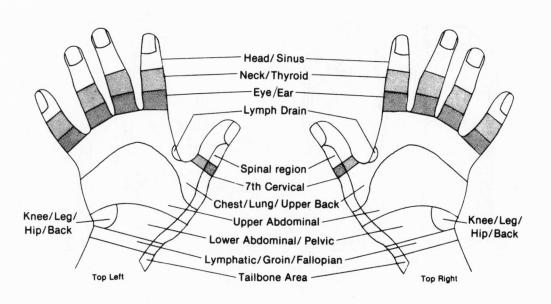

Head/Sinus

Neck/Thyroid

Eye/Ear

Lymph Drain

Spinal region

7th Cervical

Chest/Lung/Upper Back

Upper Abdominal

Lower Abdominal/Pelvic

Lymphatic/Groin/Fallopian

Tailbone Area

Knee/Leg/Hip/Back

Knee/Leg/Hip/Back

Top Left

Top Right

FOOT REFLEXOLOGY CHARTS

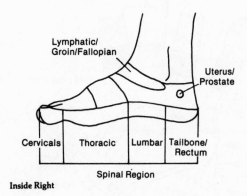

Lymphatic/
Groin/Fallopian

Uterus/
Prostate

Cervicals   Thoracic   Lumbar   Tailbone/
Rectum

Spinal Region

Inside Right

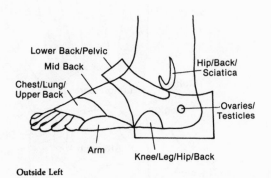

Lower Back/Pelvic

Mid Back

Chest/Lung/
Upper Back

Hip/Back/
Sciatica

Ovaries/
Testicles

Arm

Knee/Leg/Hip/Back

Outside Left

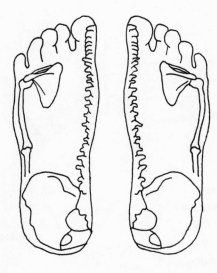

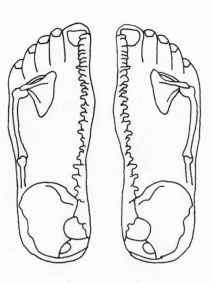

ZONE CHARTS

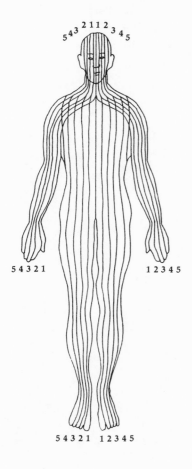

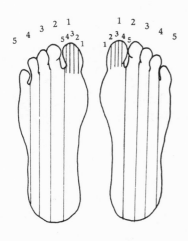

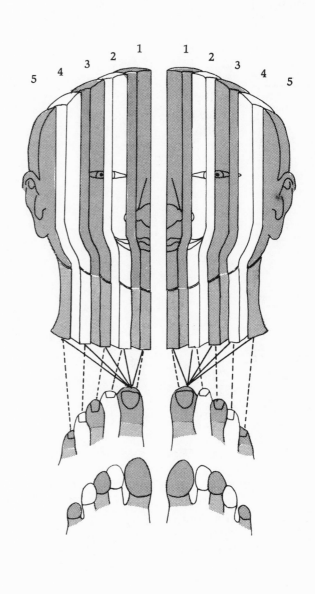

GLOSSARY OF SYMBOLS: BASIC TECHNIQUES

 Single Finger Grip (page 27)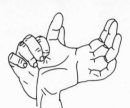

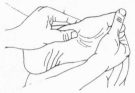 Thumb Walking (page 32)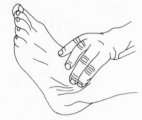

 Multiple Finger Grip (page 28)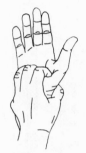

 Finger Walking (page 33)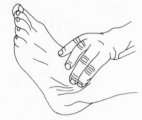

 The Pinch (page 28)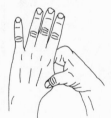

 Multiple Finger Walking (page 33)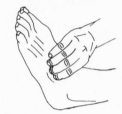

 Direct Grip (page 29)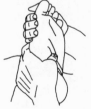

 Golf Ball (page 87)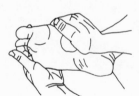

 Rotating on a Point Finger (page 30)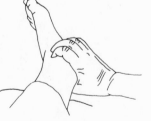

 Foot Roller (page 62)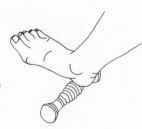

 Rotating on a Point Thumb (page 30)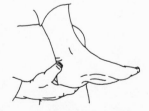

GLOSSARY OF SYMBOLS: RELATIONSHIPS

Reiterative Relationships

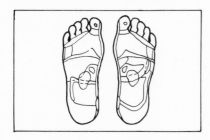 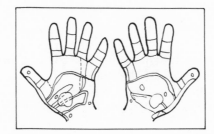

Mirroring the body whole on a body part. (See page 11) Use the chart to find the reiterative area on the hand or foot corresponding to each body part. Any area of the hand or foot is a simultaneous representation of the front, back and internal body. The right foot or hand represents the right half of the body and the left, the left half of the body.

Zonal Relationships

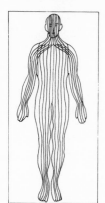

Ten equal longitudinal lines running the length of the body. (See page 11) To use the zonal relationship, begin with the reiterative area on the hand or foot or the body part of interest. Find areas of further interest by tracing the zone in which the reiterative area or body part lies.

Referral Relationships

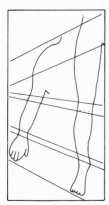

SHOULDER	—	HIP
UPPER ARM	—	THIGH
ELBOW	—	KNEE
FOREARM	—	CALF
WRIST	—	ANKLE
HAND	—	FOOT
FINGERS	—	TOES

Relating the zones using limbs. (See page 11) To use the referral relationship, see the chart to find the referral area on the limb corresponding to the body part of interest. The knee, for example, relates to the elbow through their referral relationship.

GLOSSARY OF SYMBOLS: RELATIONSHIP

Use these relationships to select reiterative areas for further assistance.

Neighboring Relationships

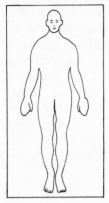

The attachment of the limb to the trunk of the body forms a special relationship to parts of the limb.
Shoulder: arm, elbow, wrist, hand
Hip: leg, knee, ankle, foot.

Relationship of Opposites

Because of movement, opposite parts of the body are related.
Neck: Tailbone
Hip: Shoulder.

Systems Relationship

There is a relationship between glands or organs in a system.

SYSTEMS	ORGANS or GLANDS
ENDOCRINE	Pituitary, Adrenal Glands, Pancreas, Ovary/Testicle, Uterus/ Prostate
DIGESTIVE	Stomach, Gallbladder, Liver, Pancreas, Small Intestine, Large Intestine
URINARY	Kidneys, Ureter Tubes, Bladder
REPRODUCTIVE	Ovary, Uterus, Fallopian Tubes (for females) Testicles, Prostate (for males)
NERVOUS	Spinal Cord, Brain
CIRCULATORY	Heart, Arteries, Veins
LYMPHATIC	Lymph Ducts, Spleen, Thymus
RESPIRATORY	Lung

Technique Pattern Charts

FOOT REFLEXOLOGY / STRIDE REPLICATION

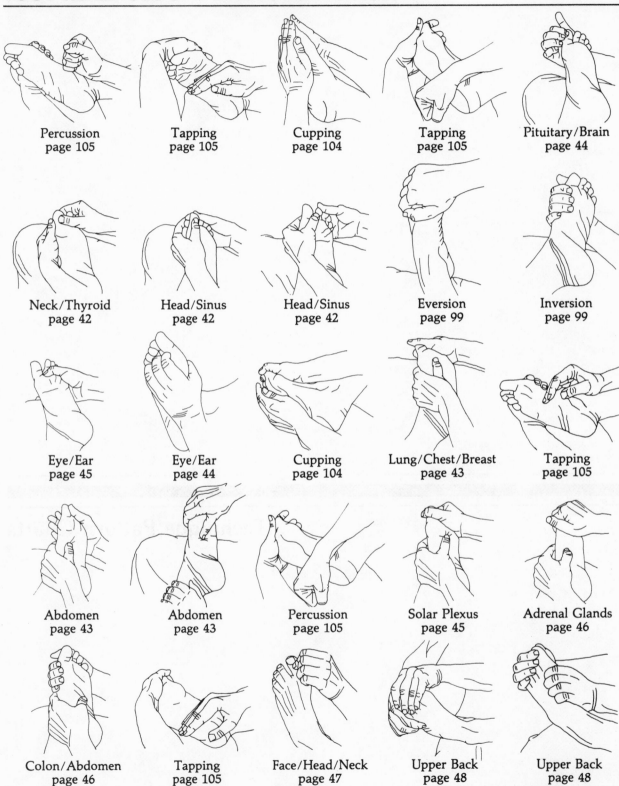

Percussion
page 105

Tapping
page 105

Cupping
page 104

Tapping
page 105

Pituitary/Brain
page 44

Neck/Thyroid
page 42

Head/Sinus
page 42

Head/Sinus
page 42

Eversion
page 99

Inversion
page 99

Eye/Ear
page 45

Eye/Ear
page 44

Cupping
page 104

Lung/Chest/Breast
page 43

Tapping
page 105

Abdomen
page 43

Abdomen
page 43

Percussion
page 105

Solar Plexus
page 45

Adrenal Glands
page 46

Colon/Abdomen
page 46

Tapping
page 105

Face/Head/Neck
page 47

Upper Back
page 48

Upper Back
page 48

TECHNIQUE PATTERN CHART

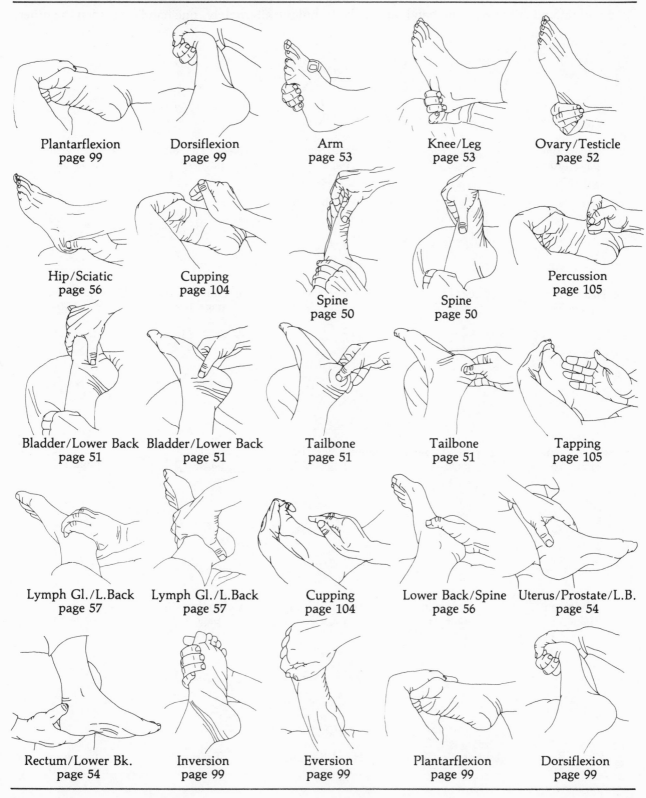

Plantarflexion
page 99

Dorsiflexion
page 99

Arm
page 53

Knee/Leg
page 53

Ovary/Testicle
page 52

Hip/Sciatic
page 56

Cupping
page 104

Spine
page 50

Spine
page 50

Percussion
page 105

Bladder/Lower Back
page 51

Bladder/Lower Back
page 51

Tailbone
page 51

Tailbone
page 51

Tapping
page 105

Lymph Gl./L.Back
page 57

Lymph Gl./L.Back
page 57

Cupping
page 104

Lower Back/Spine
page 56

Uterus/Prostate/L.B.
page 54

Rectum/Lower Bk.
page 54

Inversion
page 99

Eversion
page 99

Plantarflexion
page 99

Dorsiflexion
page 99

HAND REFLEXOLOGY / DIRECTIONAL MOVEMENT

To avoid fatigue of the working hand, apply the technique alternately, one hand first, then the other.

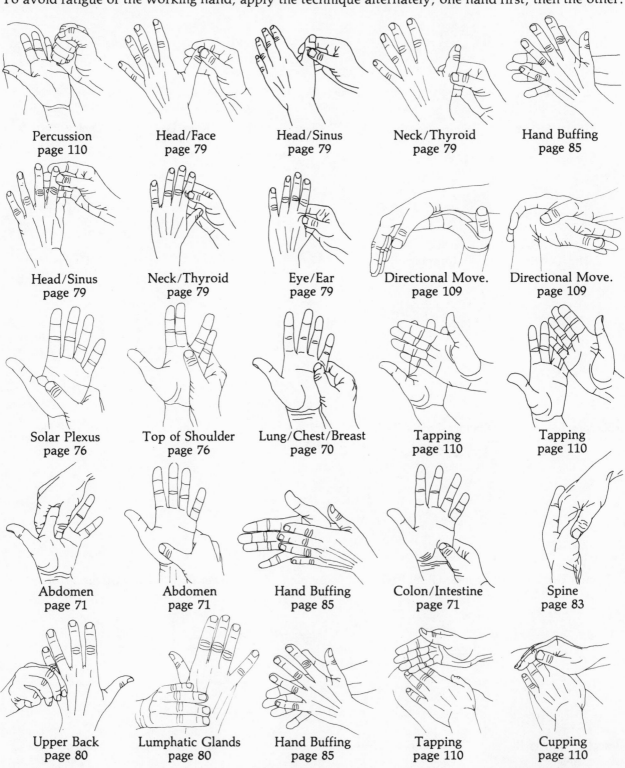

Percussion
page 110

Head/Face
page 79

Head/Sinus
page 79

Neck/Thyroid
page 79

Hand Buffing
page 85

Head/Sinus
page 79

Neck/Thyroid
page 79

Eye/Ear
page 79

Directional Move.
page 109

Directional Move.
page 109

Solar Plexus
page 76

Top of Shoulder
page 76

Lung/Chest/Breast
page 70

Tapping
page 110

Tapping
page 110

Abdomen
page 71

Abdomen
page 71

Hand Buffing
page 85

Colon/Intestine
page 71

Spine
page 83

Upper Back
page 80

Lumphatic Glands
page 80

Hand Buffing
page 85

Tapping
page 110

Cupping
page 110

TECHNIQUE PATTERN CHART

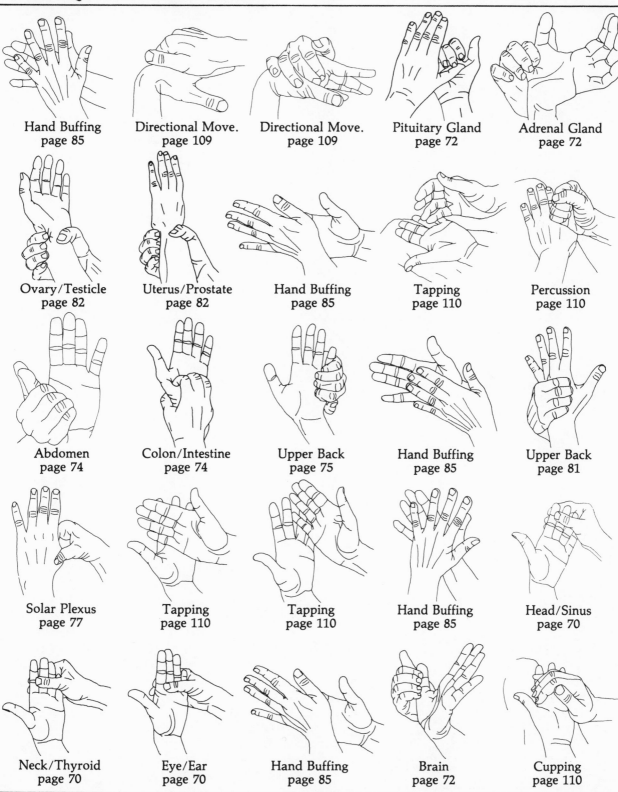

Hand Buffing
page 85

Directional Move.
page 109

Directional Move.
page 109

Pituitary Gland
page 72

Adrenal Gland
page 72

Ovary/Testicle
page 82

Uterus/Prostate
page 82

Hand Buffing
page 85

Tapping
page 110

Percussion
page 110

Abdomen
page 74

Colon/Intestine
page 74

Upper Back
page 75

Hand Buffing
page 85

Upper Back
page 81

Solar Plexus
page 77

Tapping
page 110

Tapping
page 110

Hand Buffing
page 85

Head/Sinus
page 70

Neck/Thyroid
page 70

Eye/Ear
page 70

Hand Buffing
page 85

Brain
page 72

Cupping
page 110

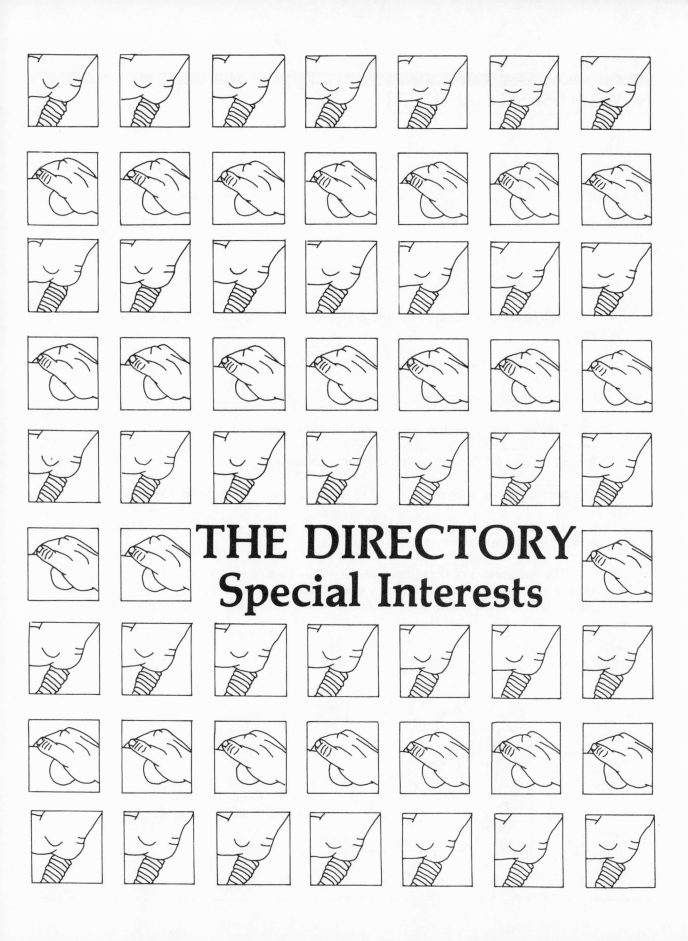

THE DIRECTORY
Special Interests

HOW TO USE SPECIAL INTERESTS

Each heading in this section provides a general description, illustrates reiterative areas.

For quick and easy reference, refer to the first block of information.

For a more in-depth look, consider all information.

The technique symbol represents the basic technique which is applied to a reiterative area. The first symbol refers to the first reiterative area shown. The second symbol refers to the reiterative area following /.

See "Glossary of Symbols", p. 115, for a listing of all technique symbols.

The "locator chart" illustrates the location of reiterative areas. See "Charts", p. 111, for further information.

The illustrations of the reiterative areas provide a reference for further information. For more information about a specific technique or other techniques which may be applied to a reiterative area, consult the section in this chapter called "Body Parts".

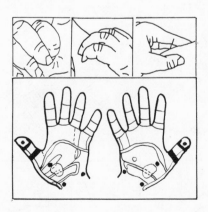

Adrenal glands, Pituitary/
Brain, / Ovary/Testicle,
Uterus/Prostate / Thyroid

ALPHABETICAL LISTING OF SPECIAL INTERESTS

ACHES, PAINS, STIFFNESS

ACNE

ALLERGIES

ANKLE (Swollen)

ARTHRITIS

ASTHMA

BRONCHITIS

BUNION

BURSITIS

CIRCULATION (Poor)

COLITIS

COMMON COLD

CONSTIPATION

CORN/CALLOUS

DIABETES

DIVERTICULITIS

DIZZINESS

EARACHE

ECZEMA

EMPHYSEMA

EYE STRAIN

FAINTING

FATIGUE

FEVER

FLATULENCE

GOUT

HARDENING OF THE ARTERIES

HAY FEVER

HEADACHE

HEART DISEASE

HEARTBURN

HEMORRHOIDS

HIATAL HERNIA

HYPOGLYCEMIA

HYSTERECTOMY

IMPOTENCE

INDIGESTION

INFERTILITY

KIDNEY INFECTION

MENOPAUSE

MENSTRUATION (Irregular or Difficult)

MULTIPLE SCLEROSIS

NUMBNESS IN THE FINGERS

OSTEOPOROSIS

PARALYSIS

PHLEBITIS

PNEUMONIA

PREGNANCY

PSORIASIS

SCIATIC

SHINGLES

SINUS

SORE THROAT

STROKE

TENDONITIS

TENSION

TINNITIS

TONSILITIS

TUMOR

ULCER

VARICOSE VEINS

WHIPLASH

Aches, pains: General body aches, pains (direct pressure)

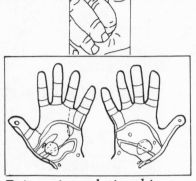 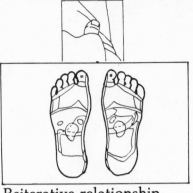 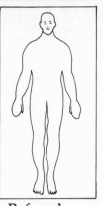 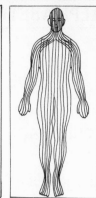

Reiterative relationship   Reiterative relationship   Referral relationship   Zonal relationship

Acne: A reaction to the stress and hormonal changes in adolescence.

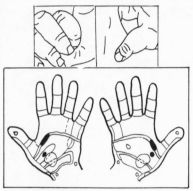 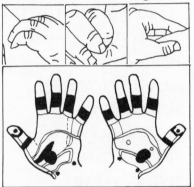 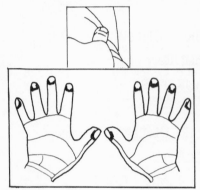

Adrenal glands, Solar plexus

Uterus/prostate, ovary/ testicle / Pituitary, brain, pancreas / Thyroid, kidneys

Face

Allergies: A mislabeling of certain food, pollen and other materials as a potential invader of the body.

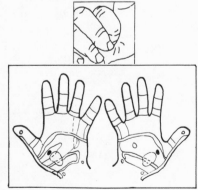 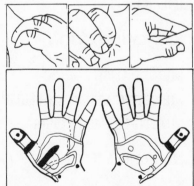

Adrenal glands

Uterus/prostate, ovary/ testicle / Pituitary, brain, pancreas / Thyroid

Ankle (Swollen, not due to injury): A failure of the body to rid itself of fluid for a variety of reasons.

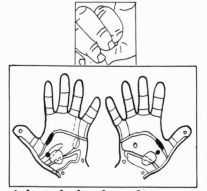

Lymphatic system, lower Ovary/testicle, uterus/prostate

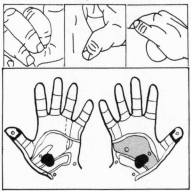

Lymphatic system

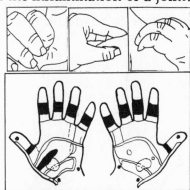

Ovary/testicle, uterus/prostate

Arthritis: A general body condition usually associated with the inflammation of a joint.

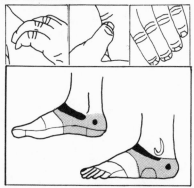

Adrenal glands, solar plexus

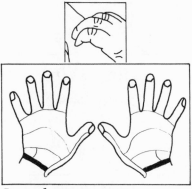

Brain / Kidney / Liver

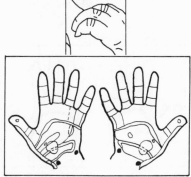

Pituitary, pancreas / Thyroid / Uterus/prostate, ovary/testicle

Asthma: An allergic condition associated with difficulty in breathing.

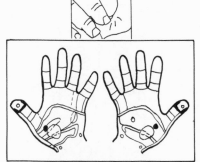

Adrenal glands, brain

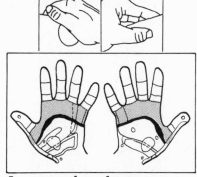

Lungs, solar plexus

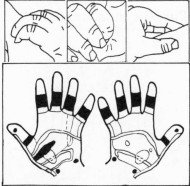

Uterus/prostate, ovary/testicle / Pancreas, pituitary / Thyroid

Bronchitis: Inflammation of the bronchii of the lungs.

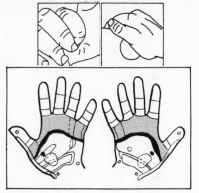

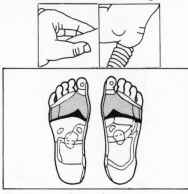

Adrenal glands / Lungs,
solar plexus

Lungs, solar plexus

Bunion: Inflammation of the joint at the base of the big toe due to irritation at the joint in response to adaptation for the purpose of stride.

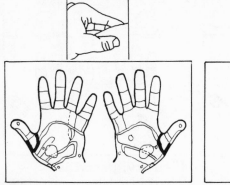

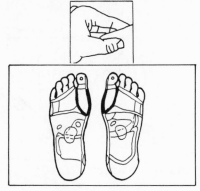

Reiterative relationship

Bursitis: Inflammation of the soft tissue sac which lies between joints.

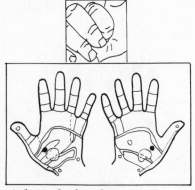

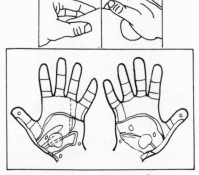

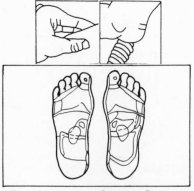

Adrenal glands

Reiterative relationship

Reiterative relationship

Circulation (poor): Interruption of flow of blood and other bodily fluids.

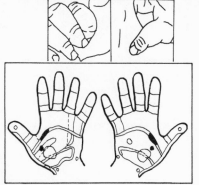

Adrenal glands /
Solar plexus

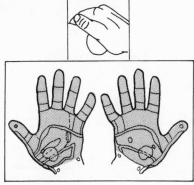

Whole hand

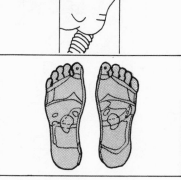

Whole foot

Colitis: An inflammation of the colon.

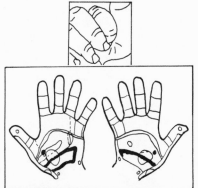

Adrenal glands, colon

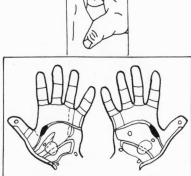

Solar plexus

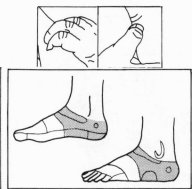

Lower back

Common Cold: Inflammation of the mucous membranes of the nose and throat.

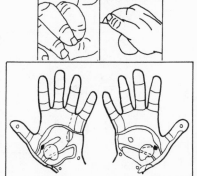

Adrenal glands

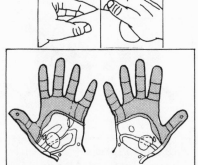

Head, throat or chest

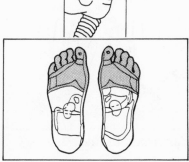

Head, throat or chest

Constipation: A condition vulnerable to the side effects of tension and lower back stress.

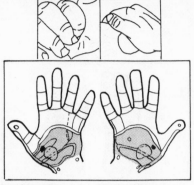

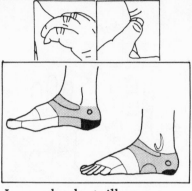

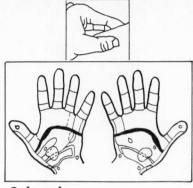

Adrenal glands / Digestive system

Lower back, tailbone

Solar plexus

Corn, callous: A thickening of the skin in response to friction or pressure. A corn additionally is an irritation at the nerve ending.

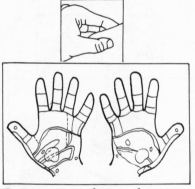

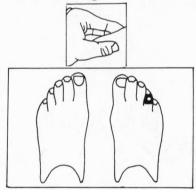

Reiterative relationship

Diabetes: The inability to burn up sugars (carbohydrates) which have been consumed.

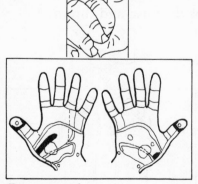

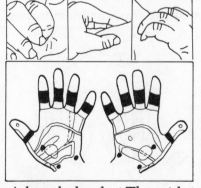

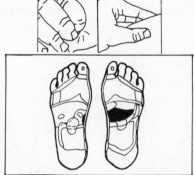

Pancreas, brain

Adrenal glands / Thyroid / Ovary/testicle, Uterus/ prostate

Pancreas

Diverticulitis: An inflammation of the colon.

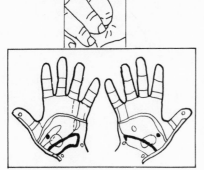
Adrenal glands, colon

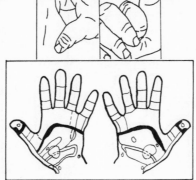
Solar plexus / Brain

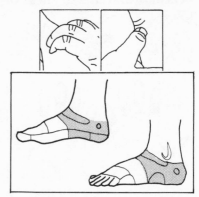
Lower back

Dizziness: A temporary loss of equilibrium.

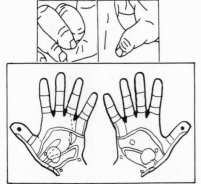
Brain / Eye/ear

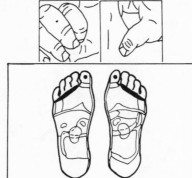
Brain / Eye/ear

Earache: Infection of the inner ear.

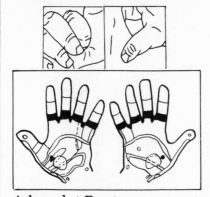
Adrenal / Eye/ear

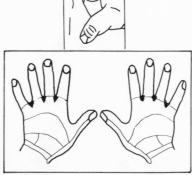
Eye/ear

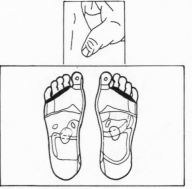
Eye/ear

Eczema: Extreme dryness of skin.

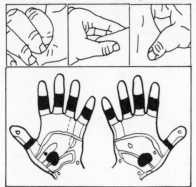

Adrenal glands / Thyroid /
Kidneys

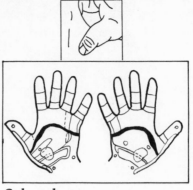

Solar plexus

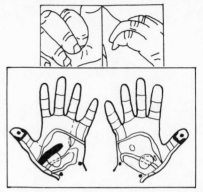

Brain, pituitary, pancreas /
Uterus/prostate, ovary/
testicle

Emphysema: Shortness of breath caused by a chronic lung condition.

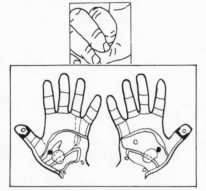

Brain, adrenal glands

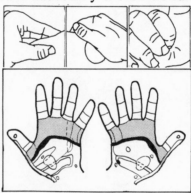

Lung/chest / Solar plexus /
Ileocecal valve

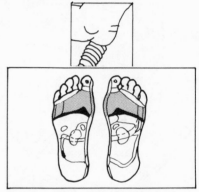

Lung/chest, solar plexus,
ileocecal valve

Eye Strain: A response to occupational, recreational or environmental factors.

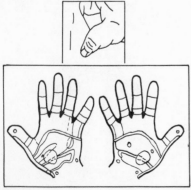

Eye/ear

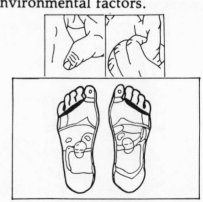

Eye/ear

Fainting: A temporary loss of consciousness.

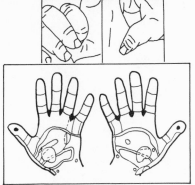

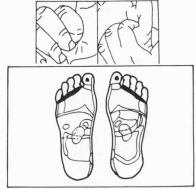

Brain / Eye/ear   Brain / Eye/ear

Fatigue: Tiredness due to over-work.

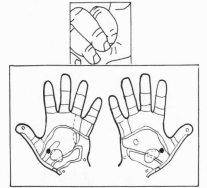

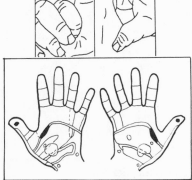

Adrenal glands   Brain / Solar plexus

Fever: An elevation of the body temperature associated with an infection.

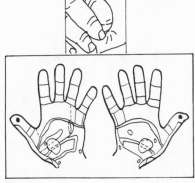

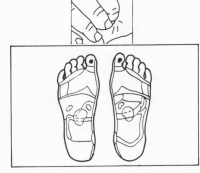

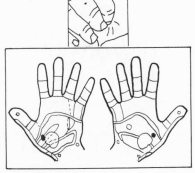

Brain   Brain   Adrenal glands

Flatulence: Excessive accumulation of gas.

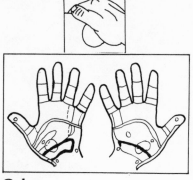

Colon

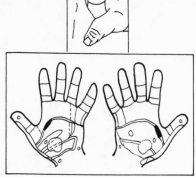

Solar plexus

Gout: Excess of uric acid in the blood causing inflammation around a joint.

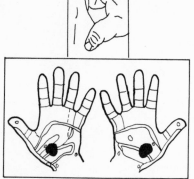

Kidneys

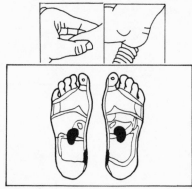

Bladder, kidney

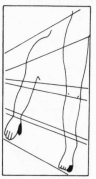

Referral relationship

Hardening of the arteries: Blockage of arteries.

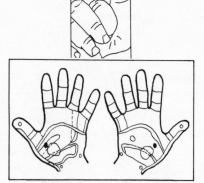

Adrenal glands

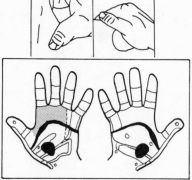

Solar plexus, kidney /
Heart

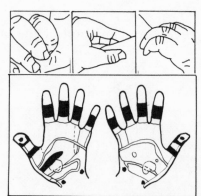

Brain, pituitary, pancreas /
Thyroid / Uterus/prostate,
ovary/testicle

Hay fever: A seasonal allergic condition due primarily to pollens.

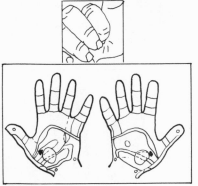

Adrenal glands

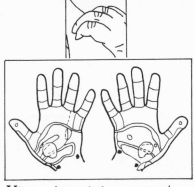

Uterus/prostate, ovary/
testicle

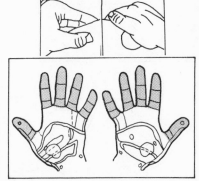

Head/neck/sinus

Headache: A response to physical conditions, stress and/or certain drugs.

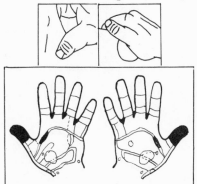

Solar plexus, eye/ear, head

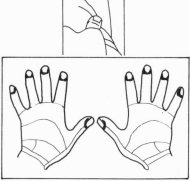

Face

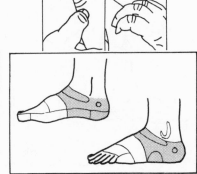

Lower back

Heart: Problems related to the heart muscle.

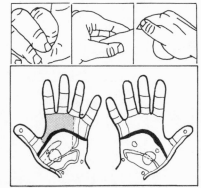

Heart, solar plexus
Brain, adrenal glands,
sigmoid colon

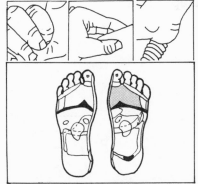

Heart, solar plexus,
sigmoid colon

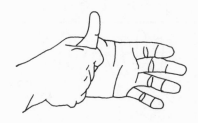

Heartburn: A back flow of stomach acid into the esophagus.

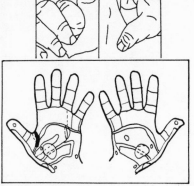

Solar plexus

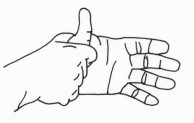

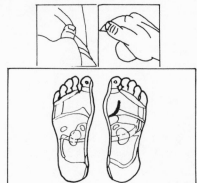

Solar plexus

Hemorrhoids: Varicose veins of the rectum.

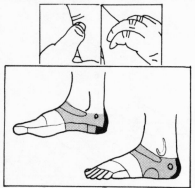

Rectum, lower back

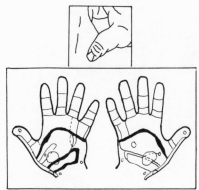

Colon / Solar plexus

Hiatal Hernia: Hernia of the diaphragm.

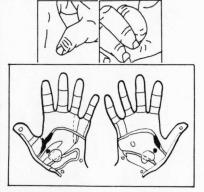

Solar plexus / Adrenal
glands

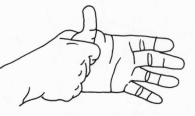

Solar plexus, adrenal
glands

Hypoglycemia: A deficiency of sugar in the blood.

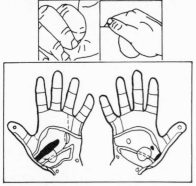 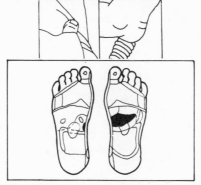 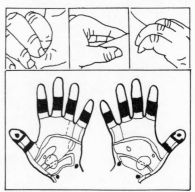

Pancreas, adrenal glands

Pancreas

Brain, pituitary / Thyroid / Ovary/testicle, uterus/ prostate

Hysterectomy: Surgical removal of the uterus.

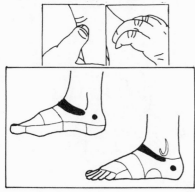 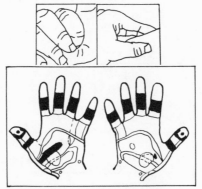

Uterus, ovary / Fallopian tubes

Adrenal glands, pituitary, brain, pancreas / Brain

Impotence: An inability to perform sexually.

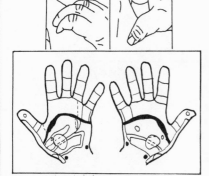 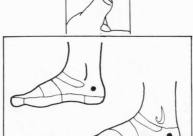 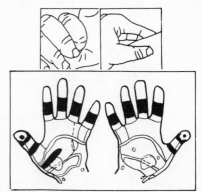

Ovary/testicle, uterus/ prostate / Solar plexus

Ovary/testicle, uterus prostate

Brain, pituitary, pancreas / Thyroid

Indigestion: A feeling of discomfort resulting from digestion.

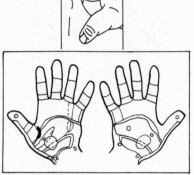

Solar plexus

Stomach, colon, small intestine

Infertility: The inability to conceive.

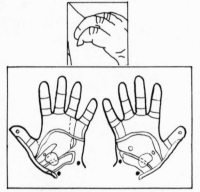

Uterus/prostate, ovary/ testicle

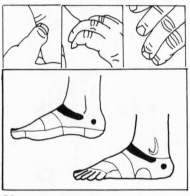

Uterus/prostate, ovary/ testicle / Fallopian tubes

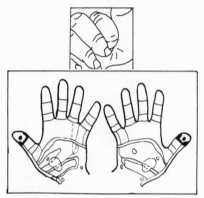

Brain, pituitary

Kidney Infection: Infection of the kidney and urinary tract.

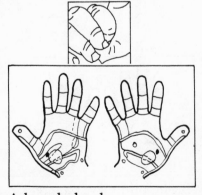

Adrenal glands

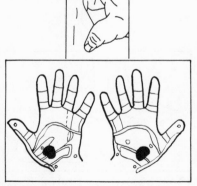

Kidneys

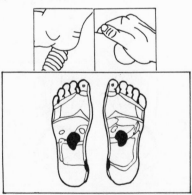

Bladder / Kidneys

Menopause: A life change in women.

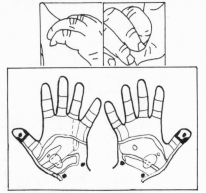

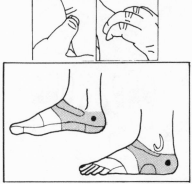

Uterus, ovary / Brain   Uterus, ovary / Lower back

Menstruation (Irregular or difficult): Periodic discharge in women of childbearing age.

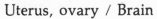

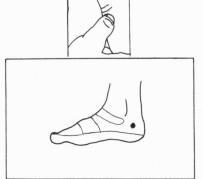

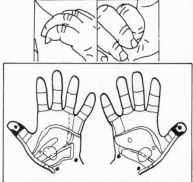

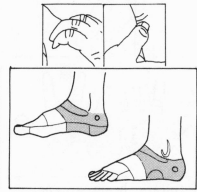

Uterus   Uterus, ovary / Brain,   Lower back
                pituitary

Multiple Sclerosis: A chronic disease of the central nervous system.

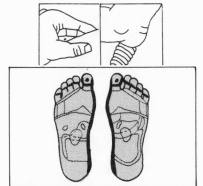

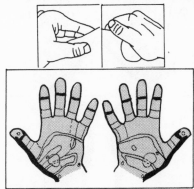

Spine, brain   Spine, brain

Numbness in the fingers: Other than normal sensations in the hand and/or finger.

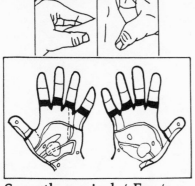 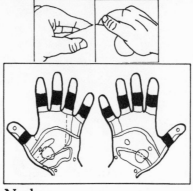 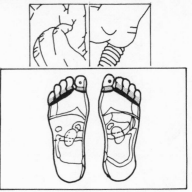

Seventh cervical / Eye/ear Neck Eye/ear / Neck, seventh cervical

Osteo-porosis: A thinning and weakening of the bone.

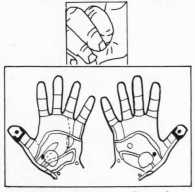 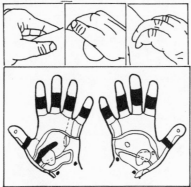

Pituitary, brain, adrenal glands

Thyroid/parathyroid, pancreas / Uterus/prostate, ovary/testicle

Paralysis: A loss of voluntary movement.

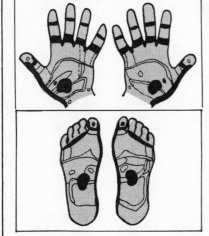 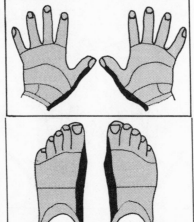

Spine, head, eye/ear, brain, neck / Kidney, bladder, entire hand

Spine, head, eye/ear, brain, neck / Kidney, bladder, entire foot

Phlebitis: An inflammation usually due to a blockage of a vein.

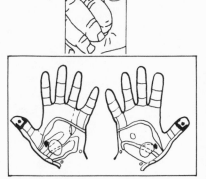

Adrenal glands, brain

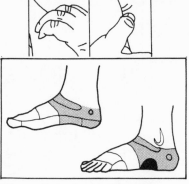

Knee/leg, lower back

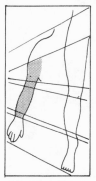

Referral relationship

Pneumonia: Inflammation of the lungs.

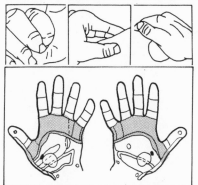

Adrenal glands / Lungs

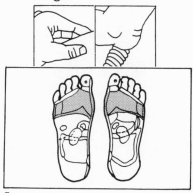

Lungs

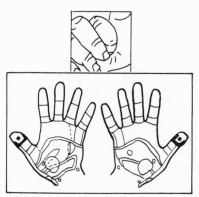

Brain, pituitary

Pregnancy:

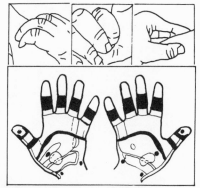

Solar plexus / Uterus,
ovaries / Brain, pituitary,
adrenal glands, pancreas /
Thyroid

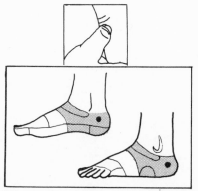

Uterus, ovaries, lower back

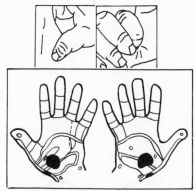

Kidney / Bladder

Psoriasis: A disorder of the outer layer of the skin.

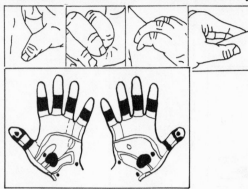

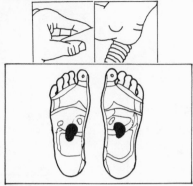

Kidney / Brain, pituitary, pancreas / Thyroid / Uterus/prostate, ovary/ testicle

Kidneys

Sciatic: Persistant pain of the sciatic nerve, the body's largest.

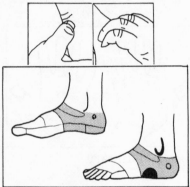

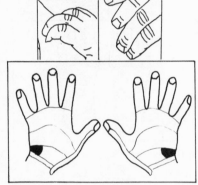

Sciatic, lower back

Sciatic, lower back

Shingles: A virus which affects a sensory nerve and results in a skin condition in the area served by the nerve.

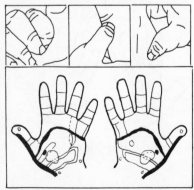

Adrenal glands / Spine / Solar plexus

Sinus: Cavities of the head which can become clogged with excessive m...

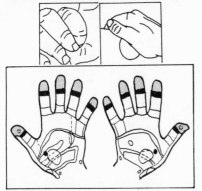

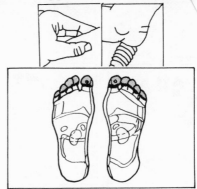

Adrenal glands / Sinus,
head, face

Sinus, head, face

Skin: The largest organ in the body.

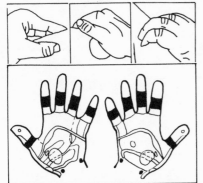

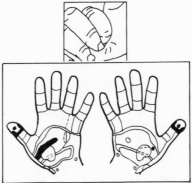

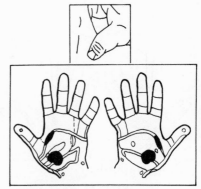

Thyroid / Uterus/prostate,
ovary/testicle

Brain, pituitary, adrenal

Solar plexus, kidney

Sore Throat: Inflammation of the throat.

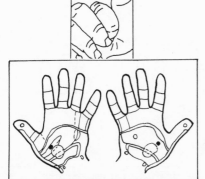

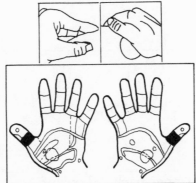

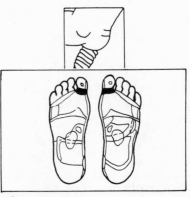

Adrenal glands

Throat

Throat

Stroke: Hemorrhage of a blood vessel in the brain.

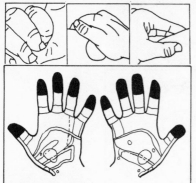

Brain, head

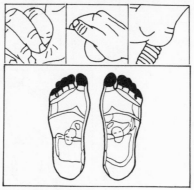

Brain, head

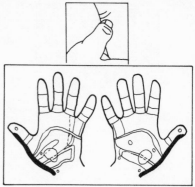

Spine

Tendonitis: Inflammation of a tendon.

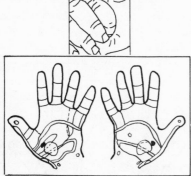

Adrenal glands

See also THEORY, Referral relationships, Zonal relationships, Reiterative relationships

Tension: Distress of the body as a whole or a body part as a result of excessive demand.

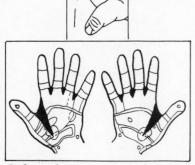

Solar plexus, tops of
shoulders

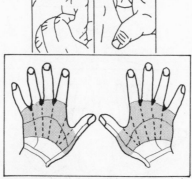

Upper back / Tops of
shoulders

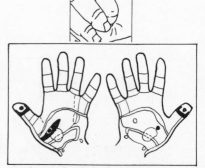

Adrenal glands, brain,
pituitary, pancreas

Tinnitis: A ringing in the ears arising from a variety of sources.

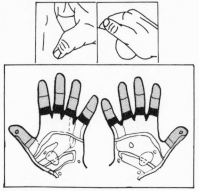

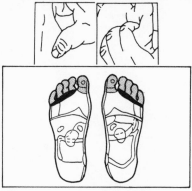

Eye/ear / Head, neck,
sinus

Eye/ear / Head, neck,
sinus

Tonsilitis: Inflammation of lymph glands in the throat.

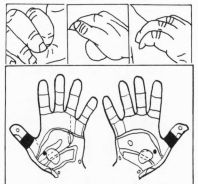

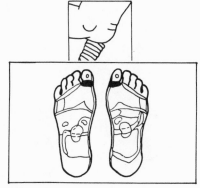

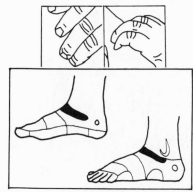

Adrenal glands / Throat

Throat

Lymphatic system

Tumor: A growth of tissue which serves no purpose.

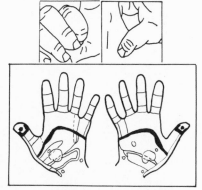

Brain, pituitary / Solar
plexus

See also THEORY, *Reiterative relationship, Referral relationship, Zonal relationship*

Varicose Veins: Abnormal swelling of veins, usually of the legs.

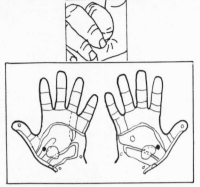

Adrenal glands

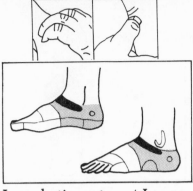

Lymphatic system / Lower back

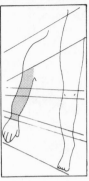

Referral relationship

Ulcer: A break in the skin or mucous membrane.

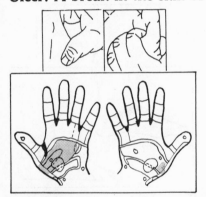

Solar plexus, top of shoulders / Stomach

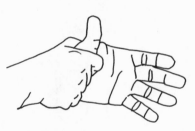

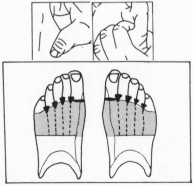

Solar plexus, stomach

Whiplash: Sprain of the muscles and tendons of the back of the neck caused by a trauma.

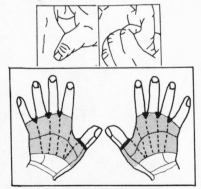

Tops of shoulders, solar plexus / Upper back

Tops of shoulders / Upper back

BODY PARTS

HOW TO USE BODY PARTS

Each heading in this section provides the location of a reiterative area and a choice of techniques with which to work. Relationships relevant to the retierative area are indicated under "Further Assistance".

For quick reference, use the locator chart and select a technique with which to work.

For a more in-depth approach, consider all techniques and "Further Assistance" as material for further application and study.

Each technique symbol represents a basic technique whose specific application is suggested in the technique illustrations. You may wish to consult the "Glossary of Symbols", p. 115, for a list of all basic technique symbols with page references to basic technique instructions.

Each locator chart illustrates the location of the reiterative area relevant to that body part. See "Charts", p. 111, for further information.

The illustrated techniques offer a selection, including those which are either quick to do, easy to learn, appropriate in a variety of settings and/or a part of a more in-depth approach. To review the technique itself, a page number reference is included.

"Further Assistance" shows body relationships of the body part. Any one or all may be combined. The potential relationships are: Systems, Zonal, Referral, Neighboring and Opposites. See "Glossary of Symbols", p. 116, for further information.

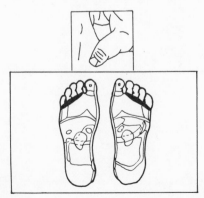

ALPHABETICAL LISTING OF BODY PARTS

ADRENAL GLANDS

ANKLE

ARM

BLADDER

BRAIN

COLON/Small Intestine

   Ileocecal Valve

   Sigmoid Colon

   Rectum

ELBOW

EYE/EAR

FACE

GALL BLADDER

HEAD

HEART

HIP/SCIATIC

KIDNEYS

KNEE/LEG

LIVER

LUNG/CHEST/BREAST

LYMPHATIC SYSTEM

OVARY/TESTICLE

PANCREAS

PITUITARY

SHOULDER

SINUS

SOLAR PLEXUS

SPINE

   Neck Seventh Cervical

   Between the Shoulders

   Middle Back

   Lower Back

   Tailbone

SPLEEN

STOMACH

TEETH

THYROID/PARATHYROID

UTERUS/PROSTATE

WRIST

ADRENAL GLANDS

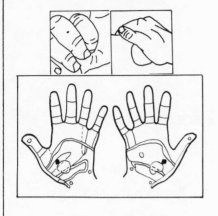

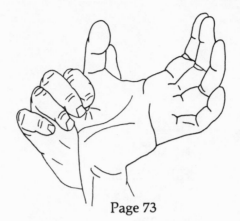

Page 73

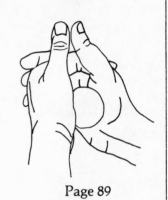

Page 89

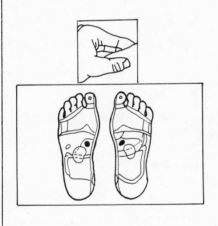

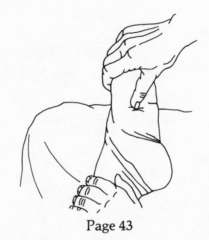

Page 43

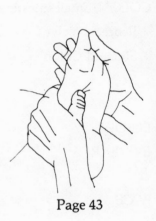

Page 43

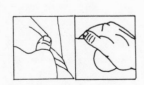

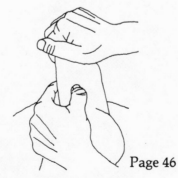

Page 46

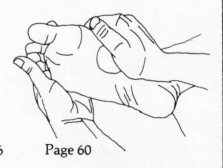

Page 60

Further Assistance:
  Systems relationship: Endocrine glands

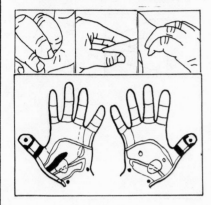

Pituitary, brain, pancreas /
Thyroid / Ovary/testicle,
uterus/prostate

Function:
One of the major
endocrine glands.
Involved in: stress,
endurance, energy,
infection, muscle
tone, inflammation

ANKLE

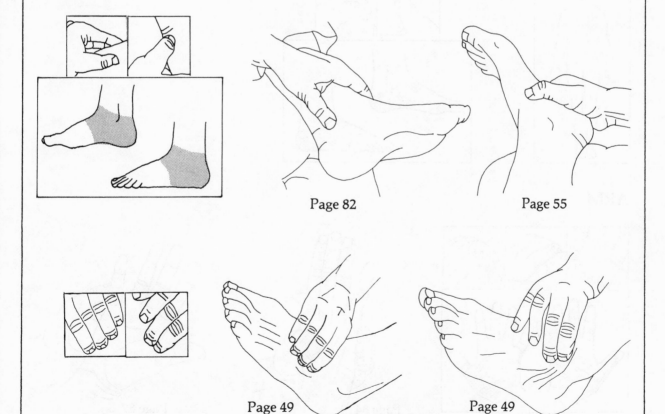

Page 82

Page 55

Page 49

Page 49

(continued on next page)

Further Assistance:
    Referral relationship: Wrist

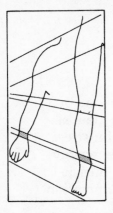 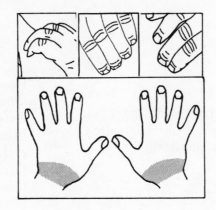 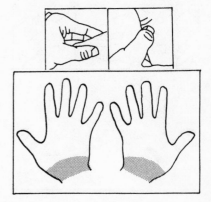

Further Assistance:
    Neighboring relationship: Lower back

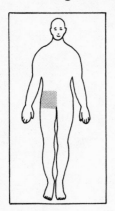 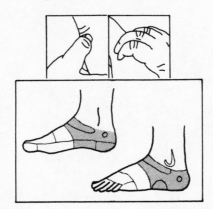

ARM

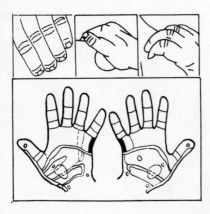 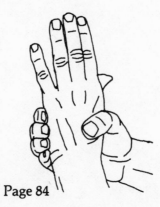 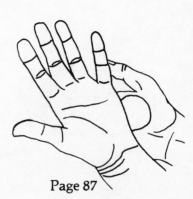

Page 84   Page 87

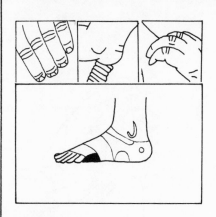

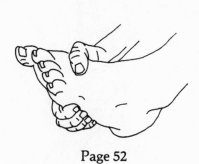

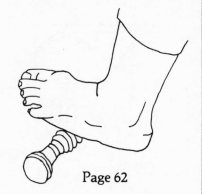

Page 52

Page 62

Further Assistance:
Neighboring relationship: Shoulder

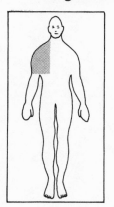

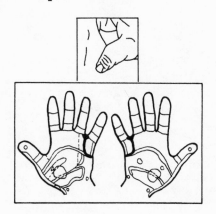

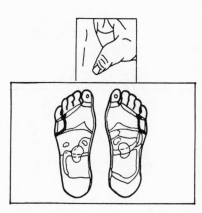

Further Assistance:
Referral relationship: Leg

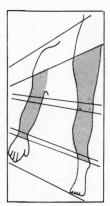

BLADDER

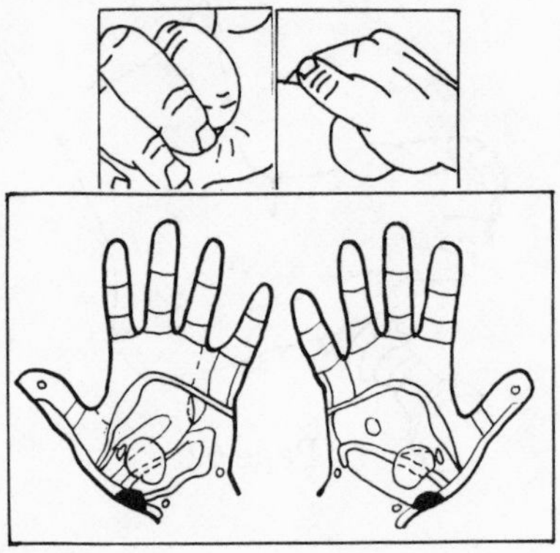

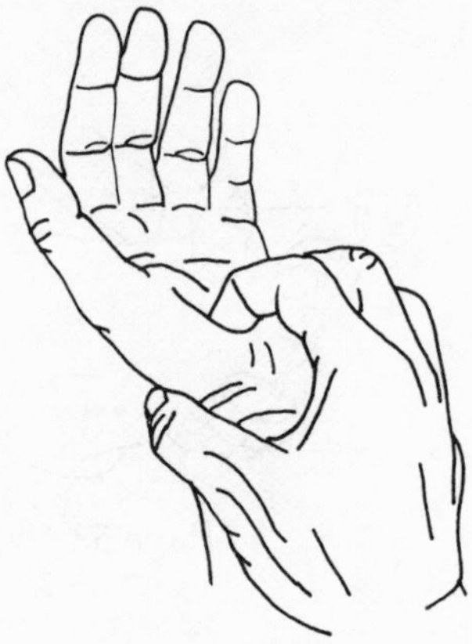

Page 73

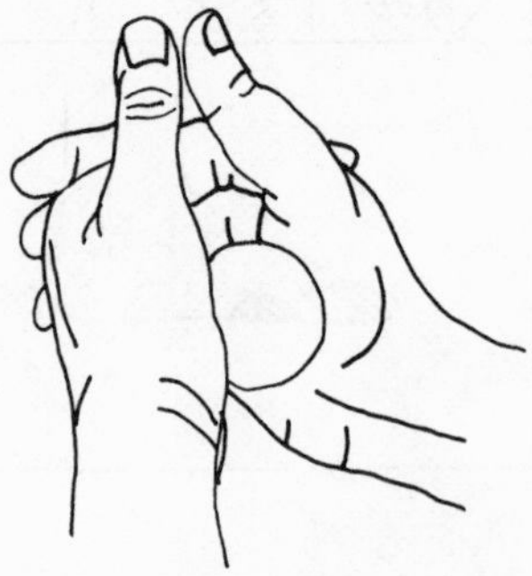

Page 89

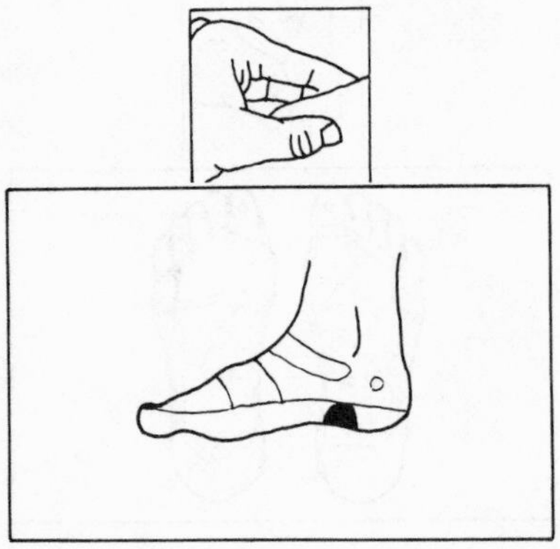

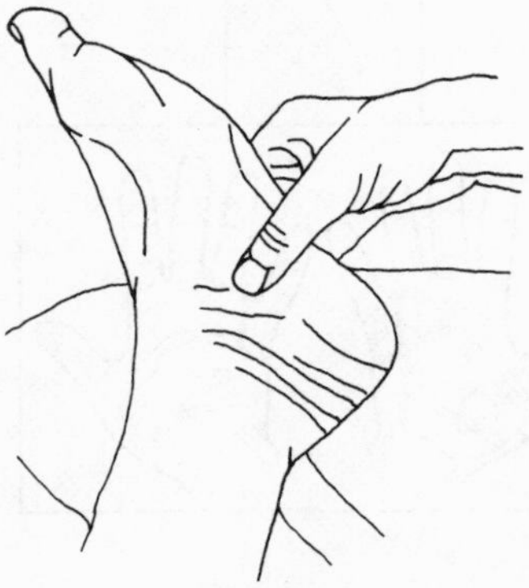

Page 51

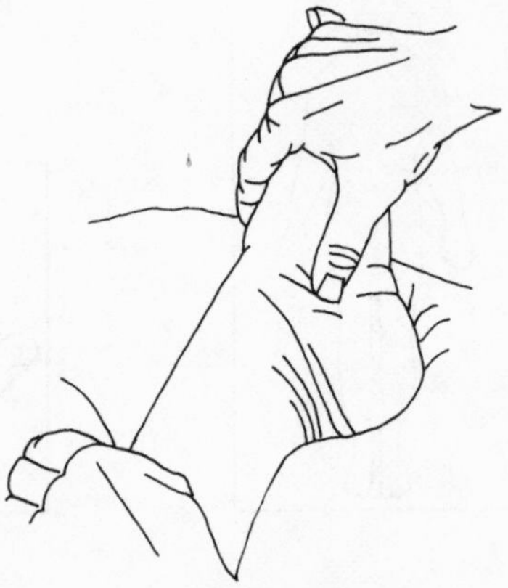

Page 51

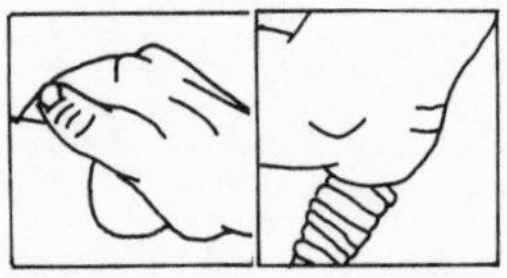

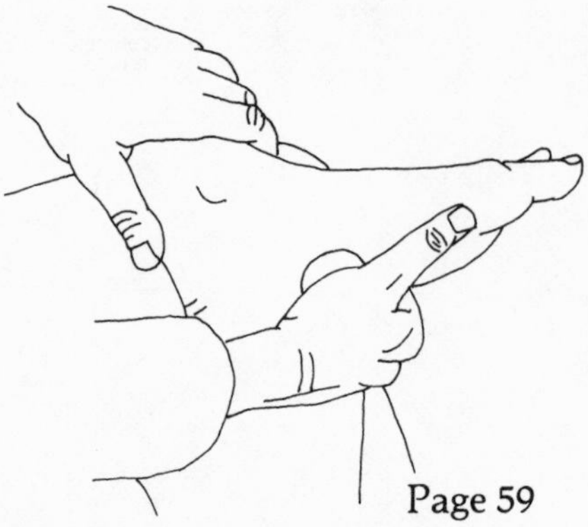

Page 59

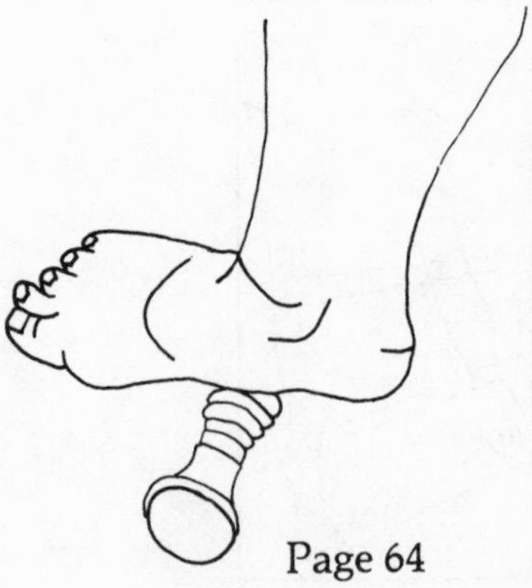

Page 64

Further Assistance:
  Systems relationship: Kidneys

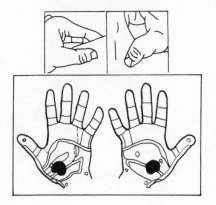

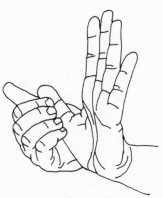

BRAIN

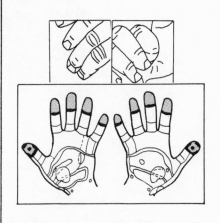

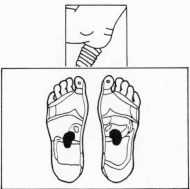

Page 72

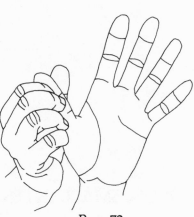

Page 72

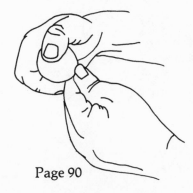

Page 90

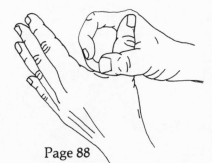

Page 88

(continued on next page)

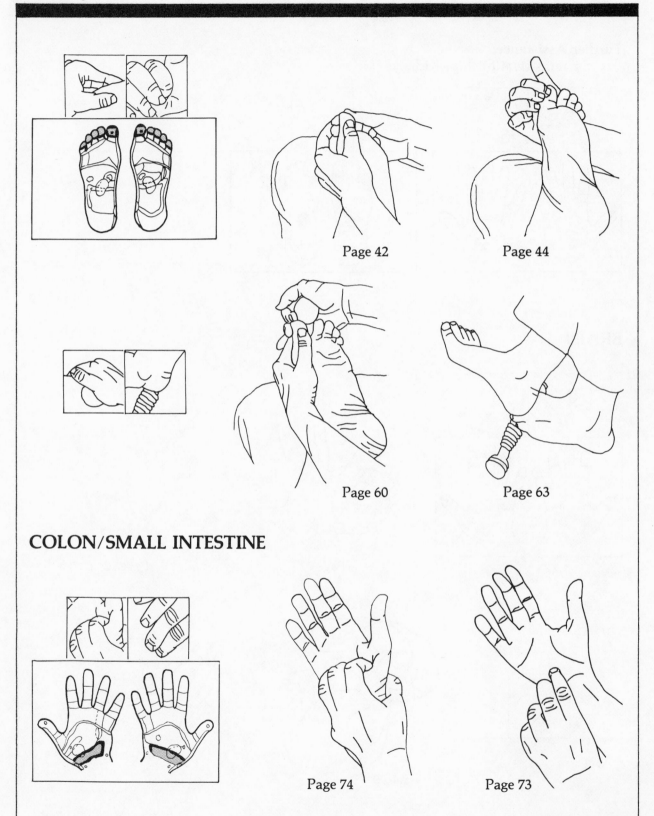

Page 42

Page 44

Page 60

Page 63

COLON/SMALL INTESTINE

Page 74

Page 73

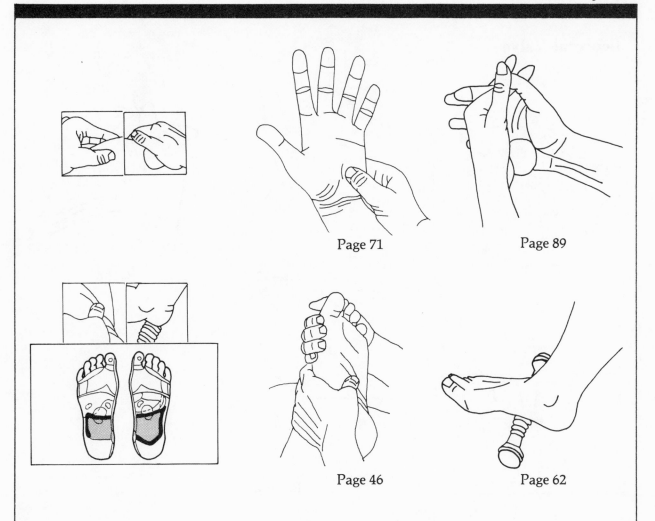

Page 71

Page 89

Page 46

Page 62

Further Assistance:
  Neighboring relationship: Lower back

Further Assistance:
  Systems relationship: Digestive
  system, Liver, Stomach

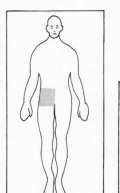

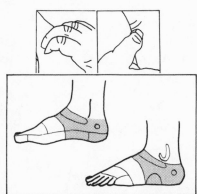

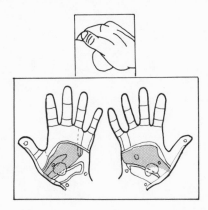

Ileocecal Valve

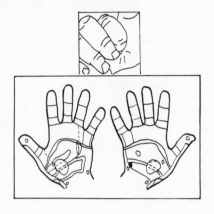

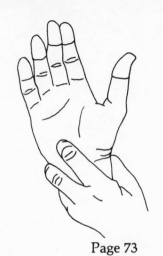

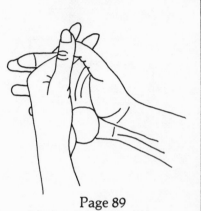

Page 73

Page 89

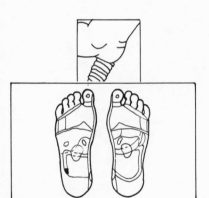

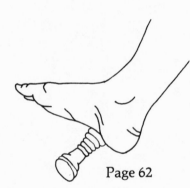

Page 62

Sigmoid Colon

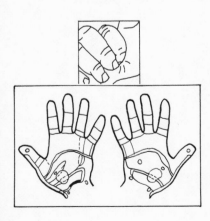

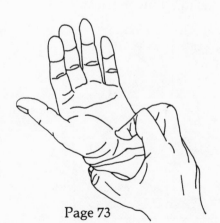

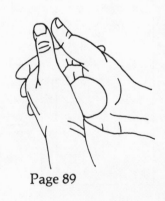

Page 73

Page 89

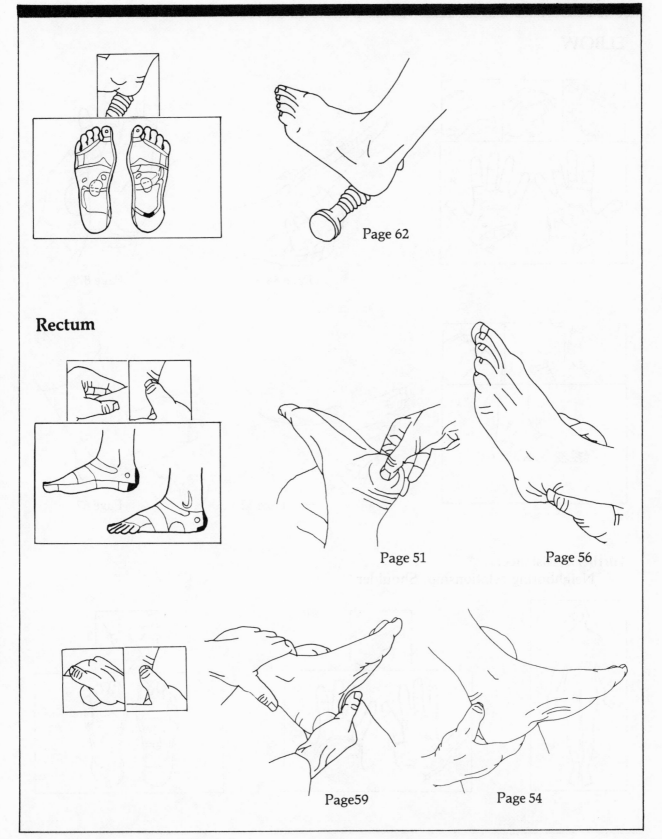

Page 62

Rectum

Page 51

Page 56

Page59

Page 54

ELBOW

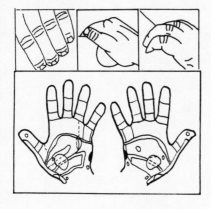

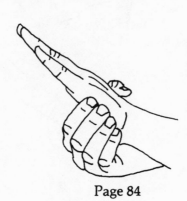

Page 84

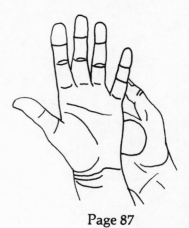

Page 87

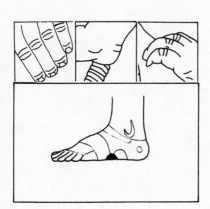

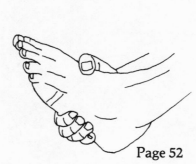

Page 52

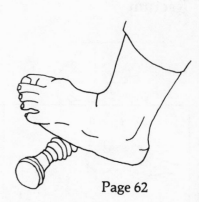

Page 62

Further Assistance:
Neighboring relationship: Shoulder

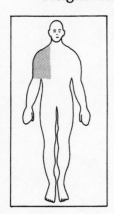

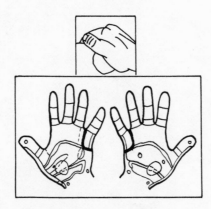

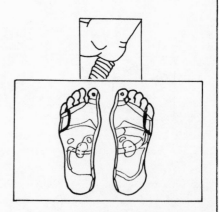

Further Assistance:
    Referral relationship: Knee

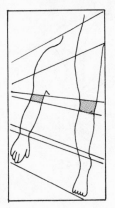

EYE/EAR

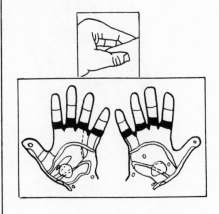

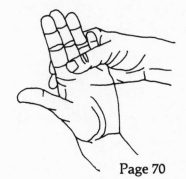

Page 70

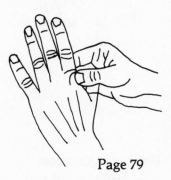

Page 79

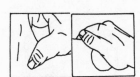

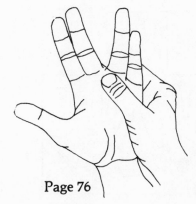

Page 76

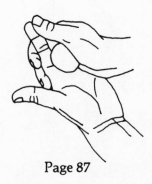

Page 87

(continued on next page)

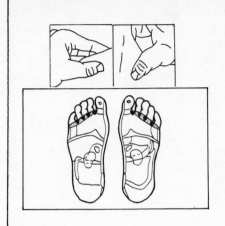

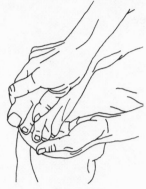

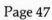

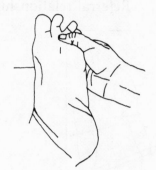

Page 47

Page 45

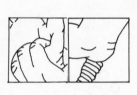

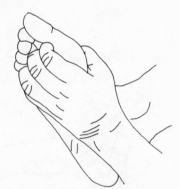

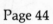

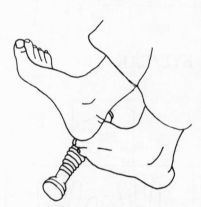

Page 44

Page 63

Further assistance:
  Zonal relationship: Kidneys

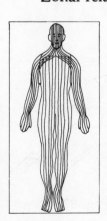

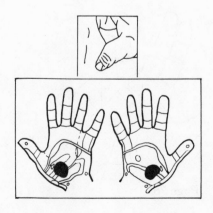

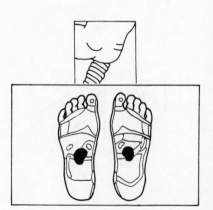

FACE

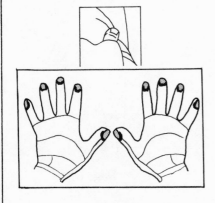

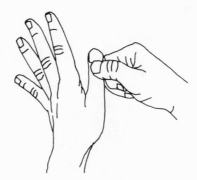

Page 78

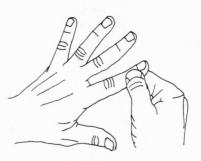

Page 78

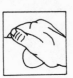

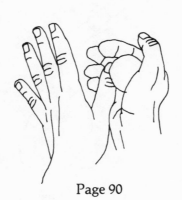

Page 90

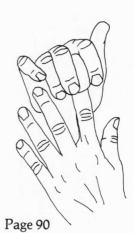

Page 90

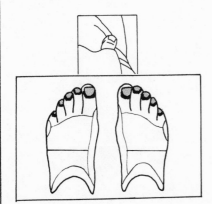

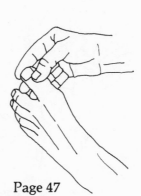

Page 47

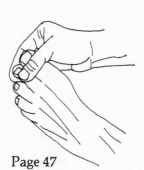

Page 47

(continued on next page)

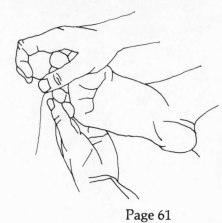

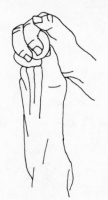

Page 61

Page 61

GALL BLADDER

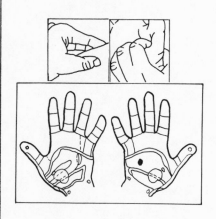

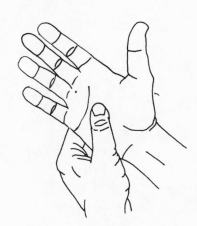

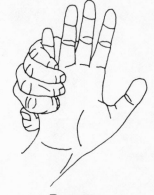

Page 70

Page 75

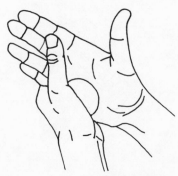

Page 89

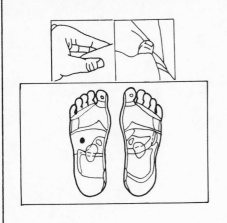

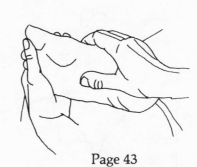

Page 43

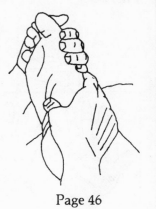

Page 46

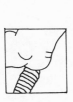

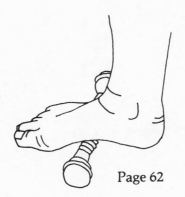

Page 62

Further Assistance:
  Systems relationship: Digestive system, Liver, Stomach

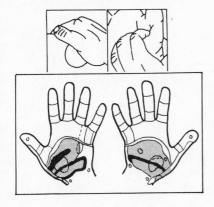

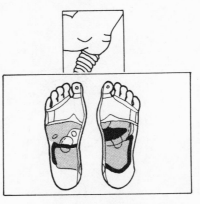

Function:
Bile storage

liver
Stomach
Colon
Small Intestine
Pancreas

HEAD

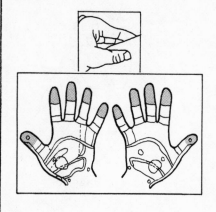

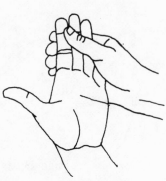

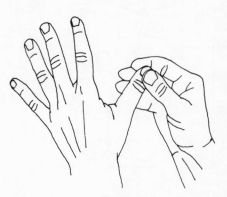

Page 70

Page 79

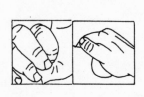

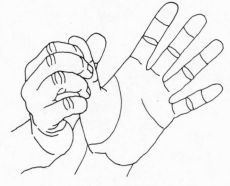

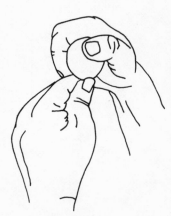

Page 72

Page 90

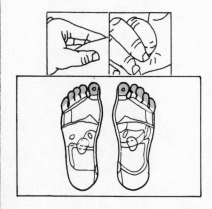

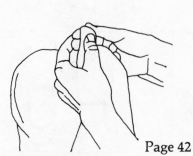

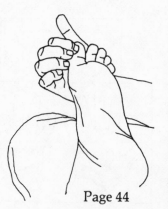

Page 42

Page 44

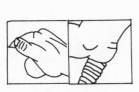

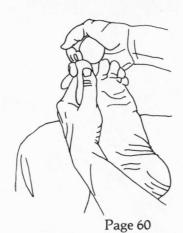

Page 60

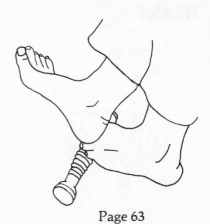

Page 63

Further Assistance:
Neighboring relationship: Shoulder

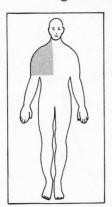

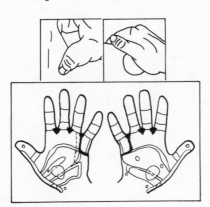

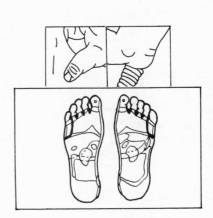

Relationship of opposites:
Tailbone

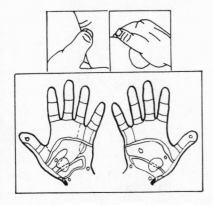

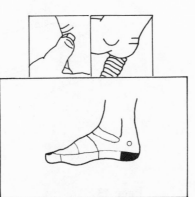

Note : Includes areas: head, brain, sinus, eyes, ears, cranial nerves, nose

HEART

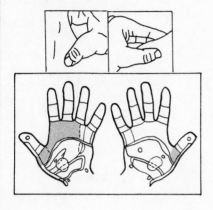

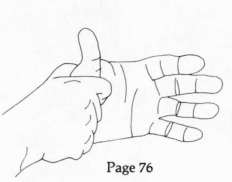

Page 76

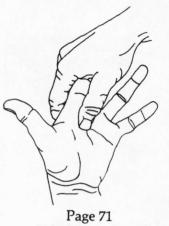

Page 71

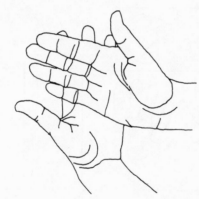

Page 110

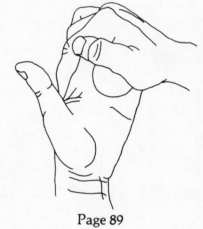

Page 89

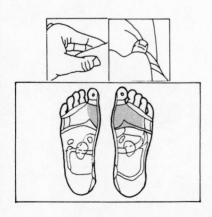

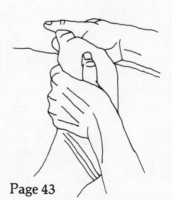

Page 43

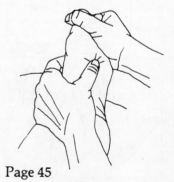

Page 45

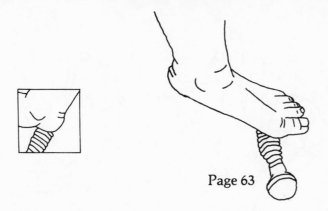

Page 63

Further assistance:
Zonal relationship: Sigmoid Colon

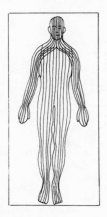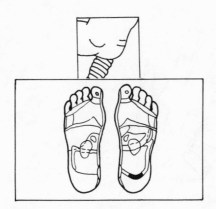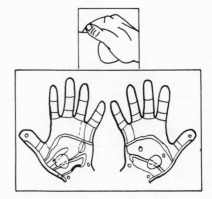

HIP/SCIATIC

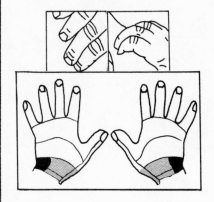

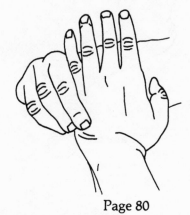

Page 80

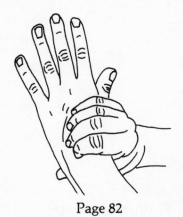

Page 82

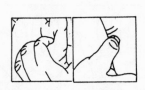

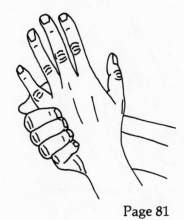

Page 81

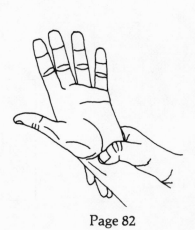

Page 82

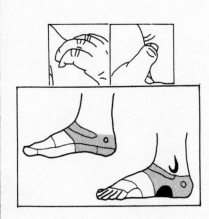

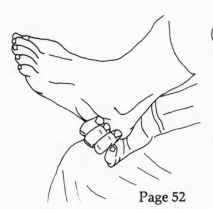

Page 52

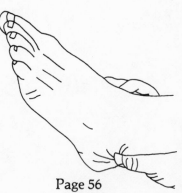

Page 56

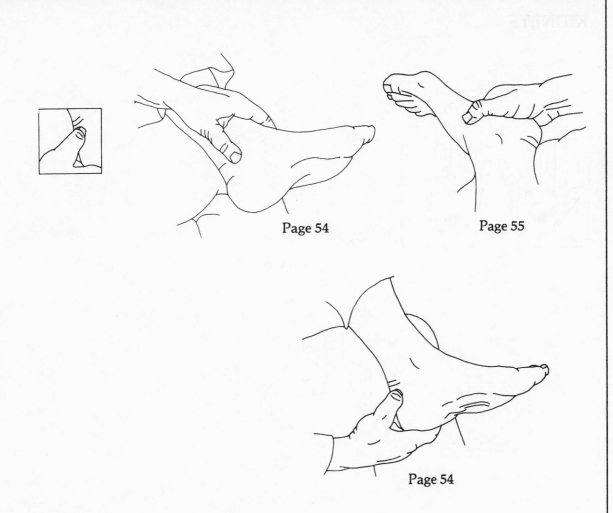

Page 54

Page 55

Page 54

Further Assistance:
    Referral relationship: Shoulder

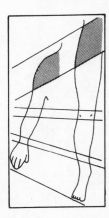

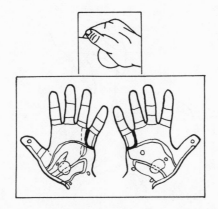

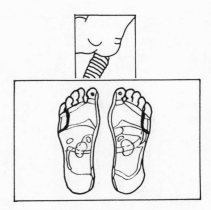

KIDNEYS

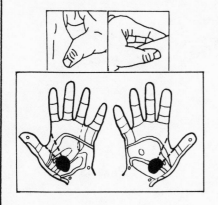

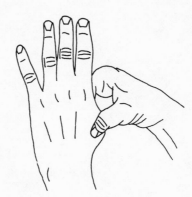

Page 78

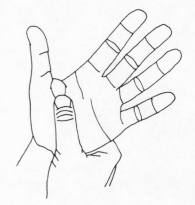

Page 77

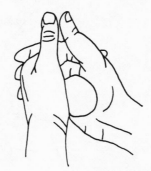

Page 89

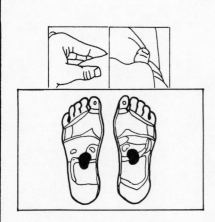

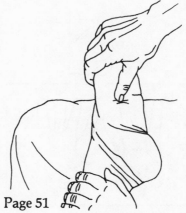

Page 51

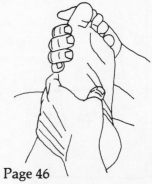

Page 46

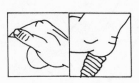

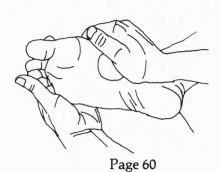

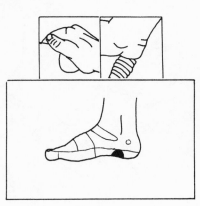

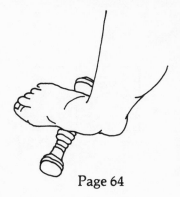

Page 60

Page 64

Further Assistance:
Systems relationship: Bladder

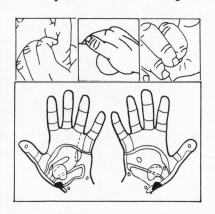

Functions include:
elimination of fluids, regulation of acid/ alkaline balance, salt, and other substances in the blood

KNEE/LEG

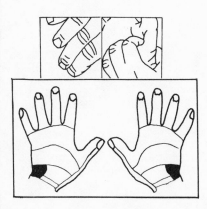

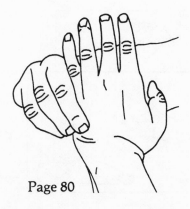

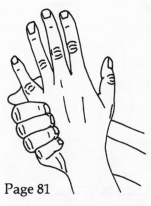

Page 80

Page 81

(continued on next page)

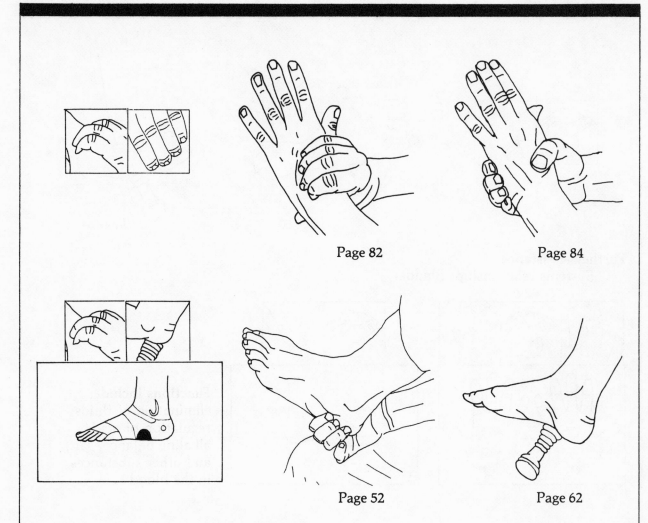

Page 82

Page 84

Page 52

Page 62

Further Assistance:
Neighboring relationship: Lower back

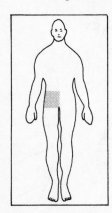

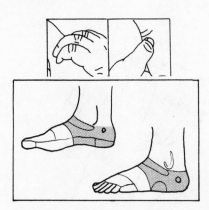

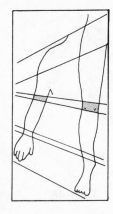

Further Assistance:
 Referral relationship: Elbow

LIVER

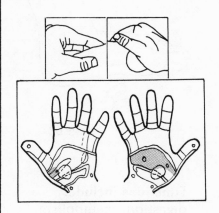

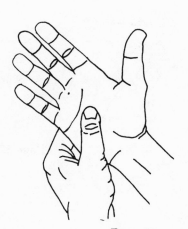

Page 71

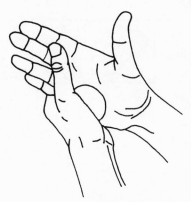

Page 89

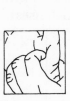

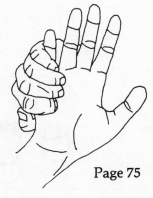

Page 75

(continued on next page)

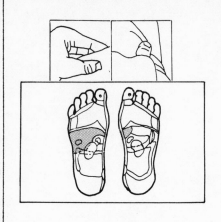

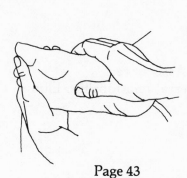

Page 43

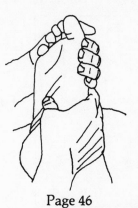

Page 46

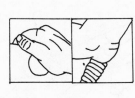

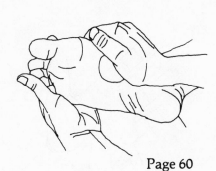

Page 60

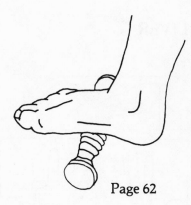

Page 62

Functions include:
digestion, metabolism, clotting mechanism, detoxifier of blood, storage of nutrients, production of body heat, contributor to the body's defenses

Further Assistance:
Systems relationship: Digestive system

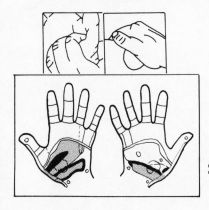

Stomach
Pancreas
Gall Bladder
Colon
Small Intestine

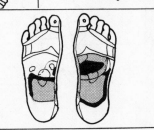

LUNG/CHEST/BREAST

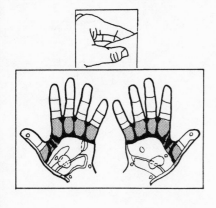

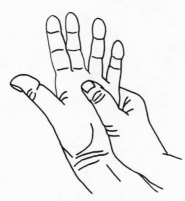

Page 70

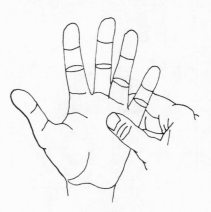

Page 70

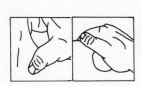

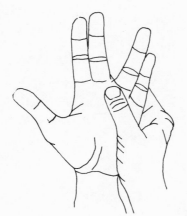

Page 76

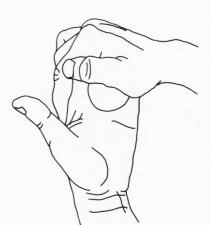

Page 88

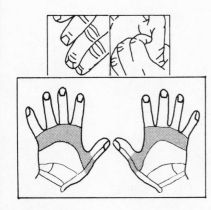

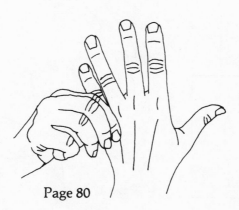

Page 80

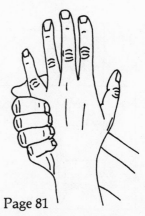

Page 81

(continued on next page)

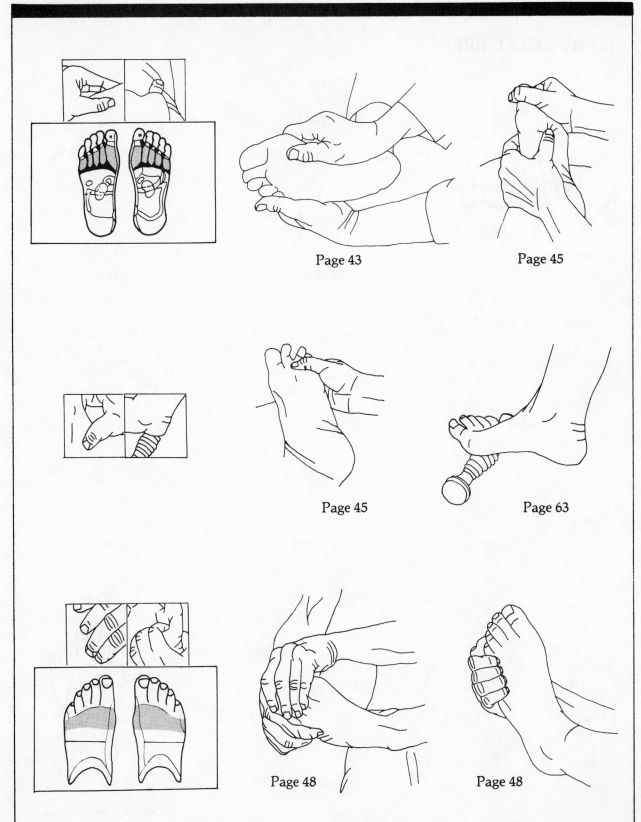

Page 43

Page 45

Page 45

Page 63

Page 48

Page 48

Further Assistance:
Systems relationship: Breast; Lymphatic System

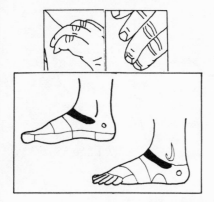

LYMPHATIC SYSTEM

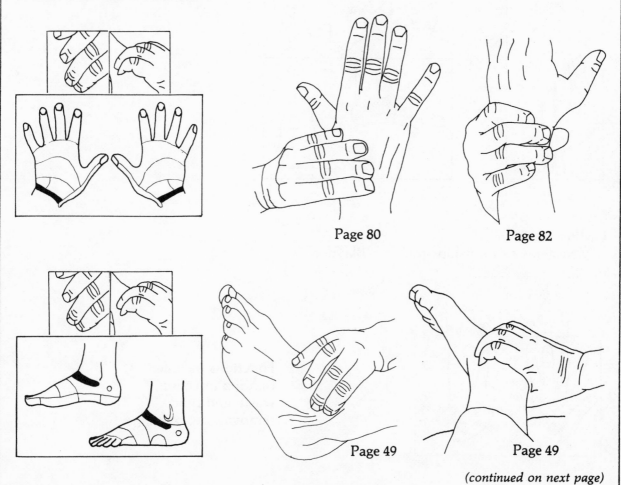

Page 80

Page 82

Page 49

Page 49

(continued on next page)

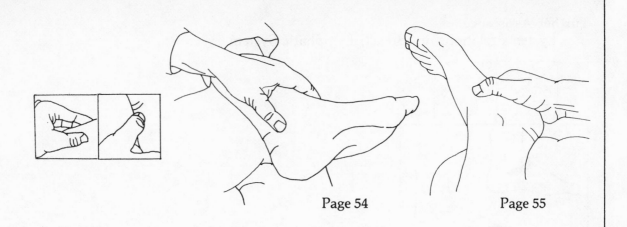

Page 54   Page 55

Further Assistance:
Neighboring relationship: Lower back

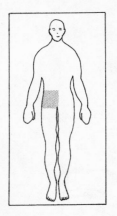 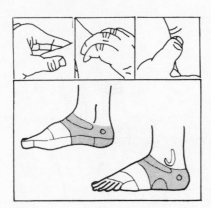

Further Assistance:
Systems relationship: Kidneys/Bladder

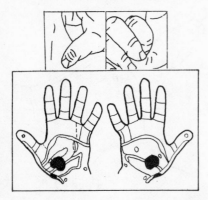

Functions include:
fighting infection,
waste and fluid
removal, detoxifying

OVARY/TESTICLE

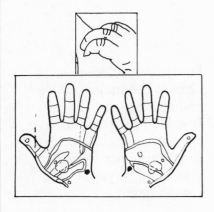

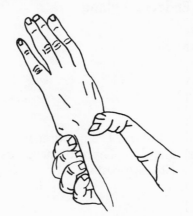

Page 82

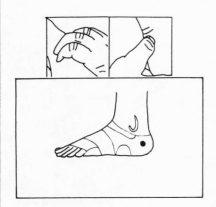

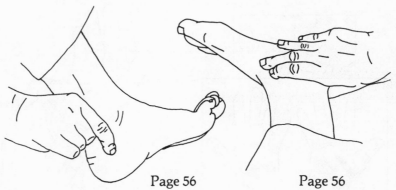

Page 56   Page 56

Further Assistance:
   Neighboring relationship: Lower back

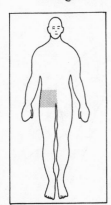

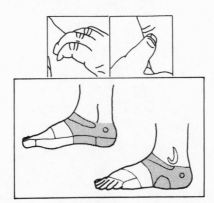

(continued on next page)

Further Assistance:
Systems relationship: Endocrine glands

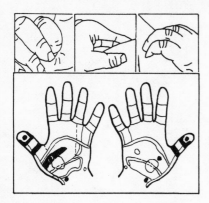

Pituitary, brain, adrenal glands / Thyroid, pancreas / Uterus/prostate

Functions include:
One of the major endocrine glands.
Involved in: reproductive capacities, maintain sexual urge, influence mental vigor and physical development

PANCREAS

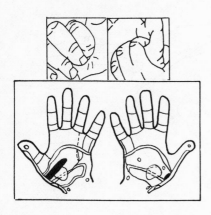

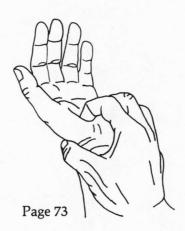

Page 73

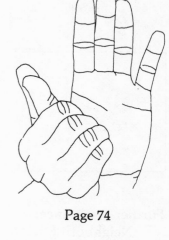

Page 74

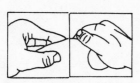

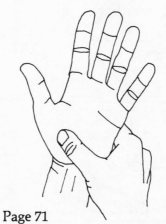

Page 71

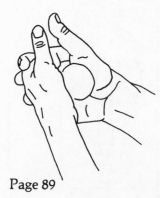

Page 89

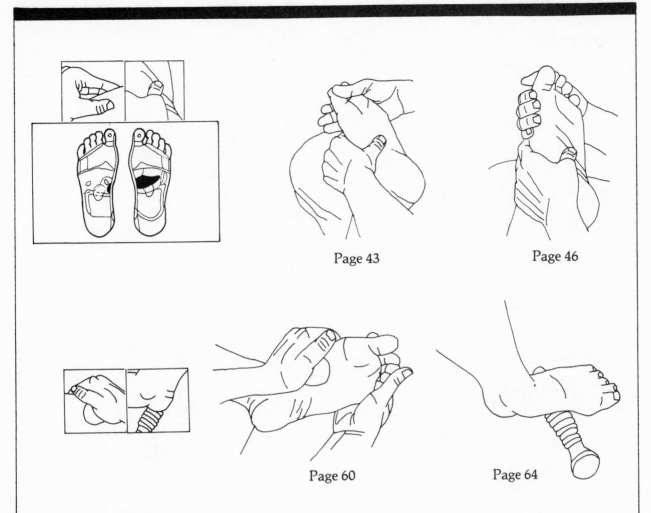

Page 43

Page 46

Page 60

Page 64

Further Assistance:
　Systems relationship: Endocrine glands

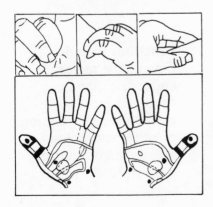

Pituitary, brain, adrenal
glands / Ovary/testicle,
uterus/prostate / Thyroid

Functions include:
One of the major
endocrine glands.
Involved in: energy,
blood sugar levels,
mental alertness

PITUITARY

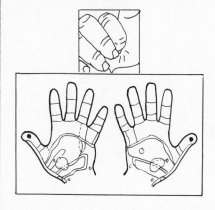

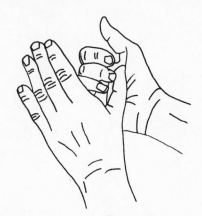

Page 72

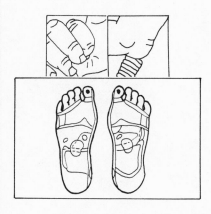

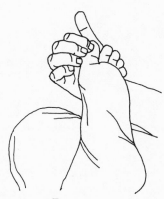

Page 44

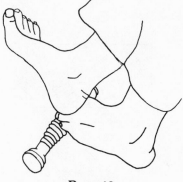

Page 63

Further Assistance:
Systems relationship: Endocrine glands

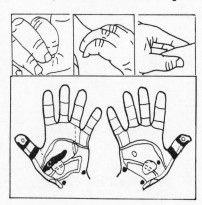

Brain, adrenal glands,
pancreas / Ovary/testicle,
uterus/prostate / Thyroid

Functions include:
One of the major
endocrine glands.
Involved in: growth,
metabolism, regulation
of other endocrine
glands, regulation of
temperature

Prostate *(See Uterus/Prostate)*

SHOULDER

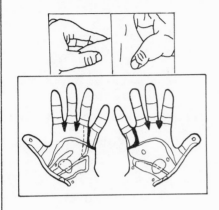

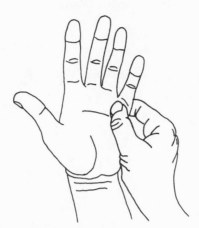

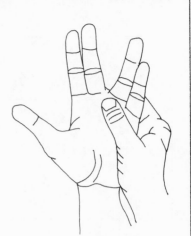

Page 70

Page 76

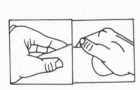

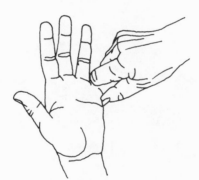

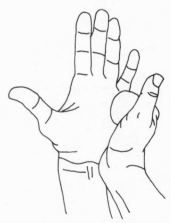

Page 83

Page 88

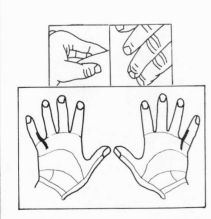

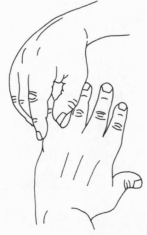

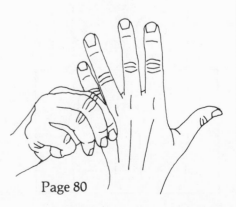

Page 80

Page 83

(continued on next page)

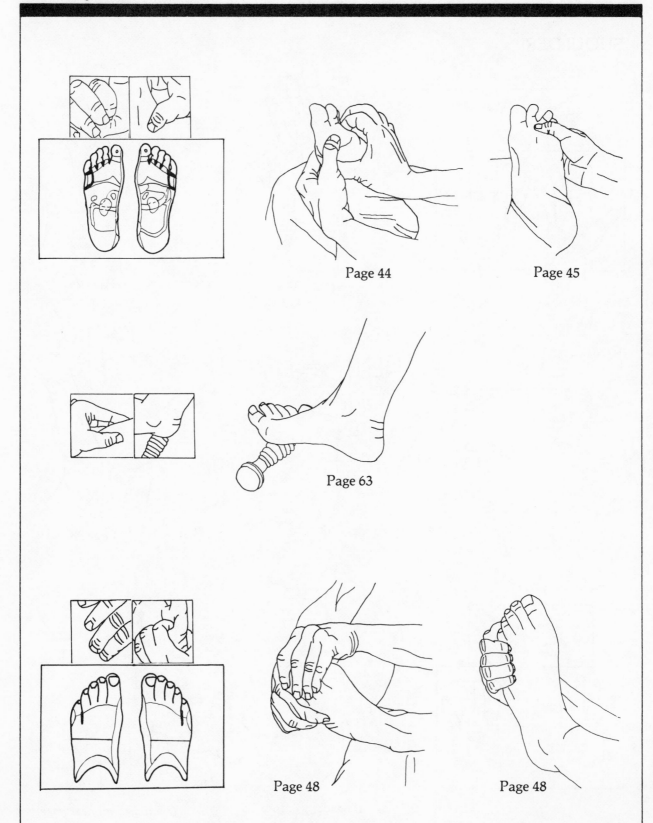

Page 44

Page 45

Page 63

Page 48

Page 48

Further Assistance:
Referral relationship: Hip

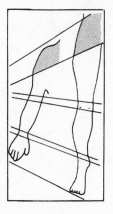

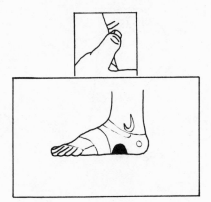

SINUS

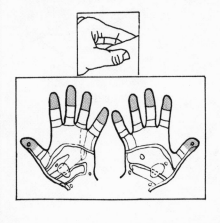

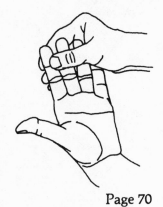

Page 70

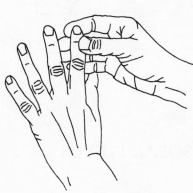

Page 79

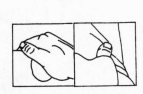

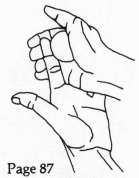

Page 87

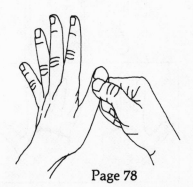

Page 78

(continued on next page)

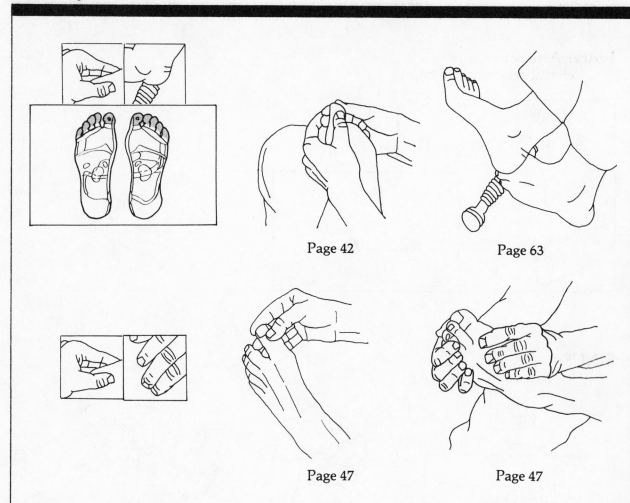

Page 42

Page 63

Page 47

Page 47

SOLAR PLEXUS

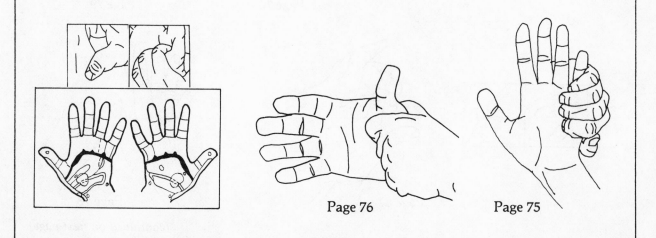

Page 76

Page 75

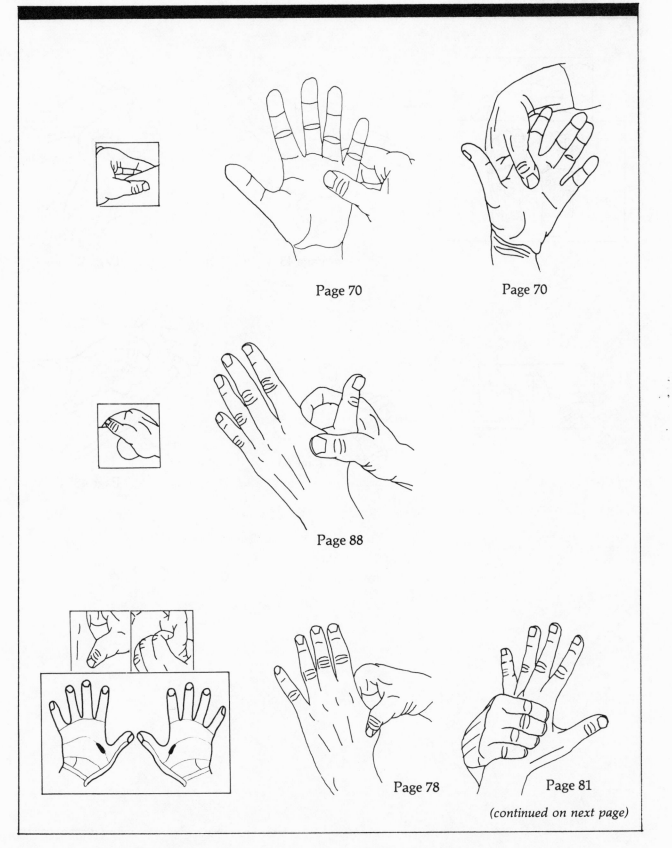

Page 70

Page 70

Page 88

Page 78

Page 81

(continued on next page)

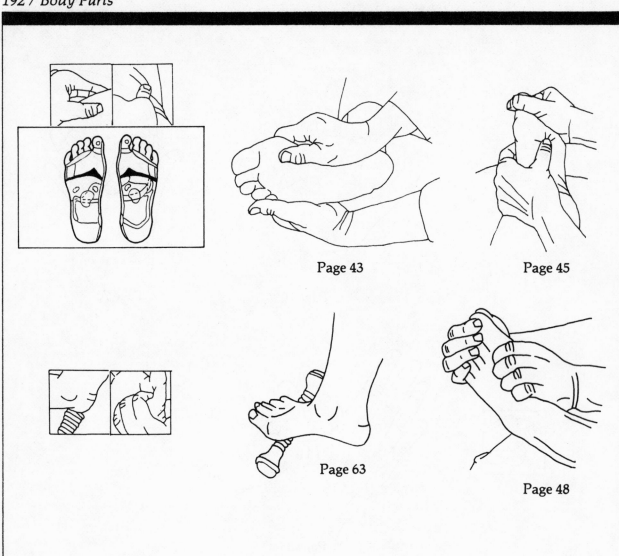

Page 43

Page 45

Page 63

Page 48

SPINE — Neck/Seventh Cervical

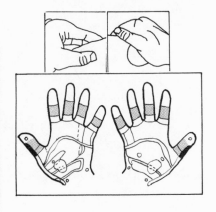

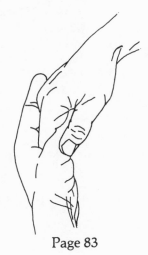

Page 83

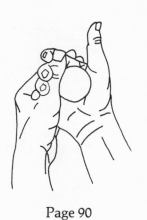

Page 90

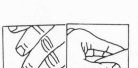

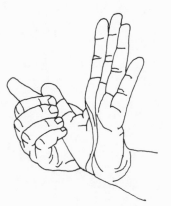

Page 72

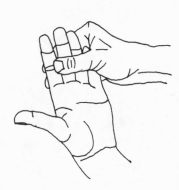

Page 70

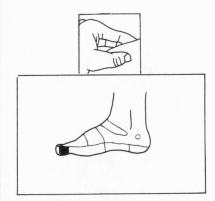

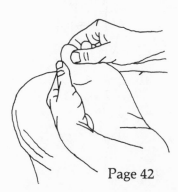

Page 42

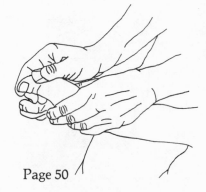

Page 50

(continued on next page)

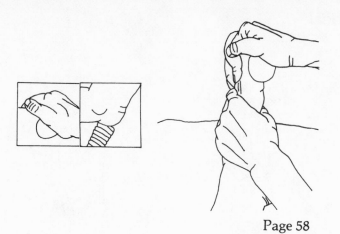

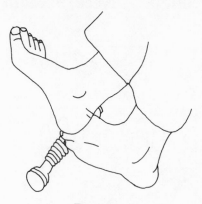

Page 58

Page 63

Between the Shoulders

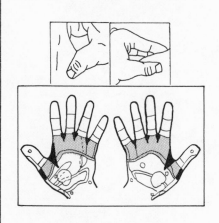

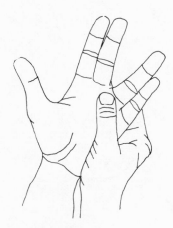
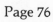

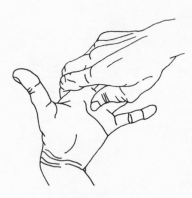
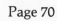

Page 76

Page 70

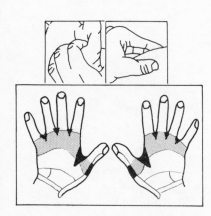

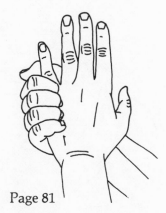

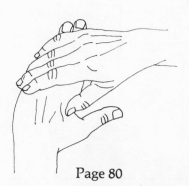

Page 81

Page 80

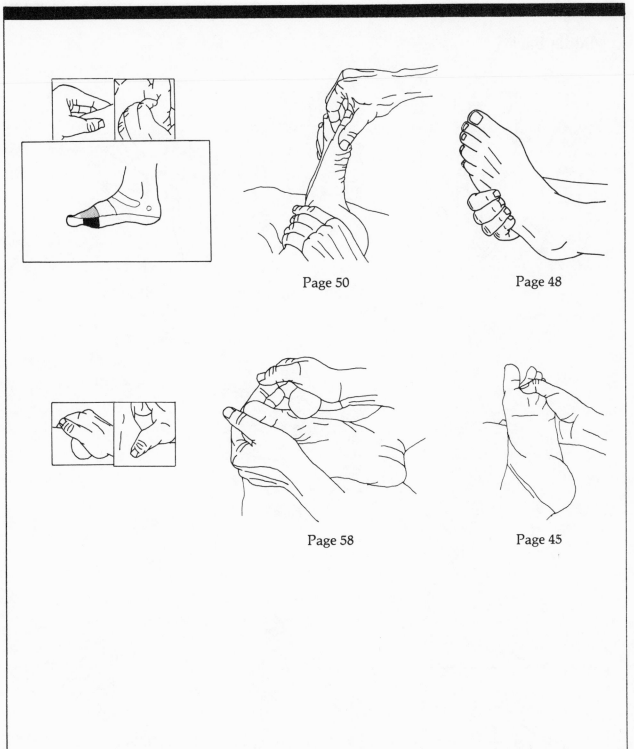

Page 50

Page 48

Page 58

Page 45

(continued on next page)

Middle Back

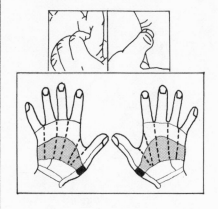

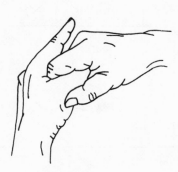

Page 81

Page 83

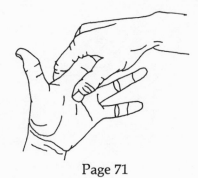

Page 71

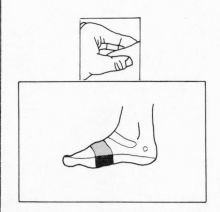

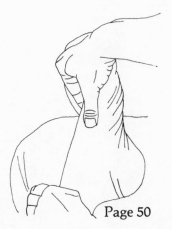

Page 50

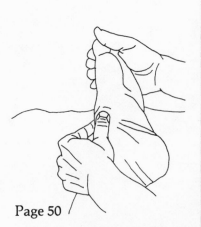

Page 50

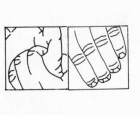

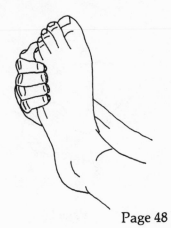

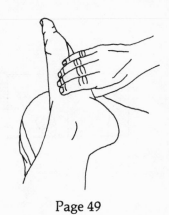

Page 48

Page 49

Lower Back

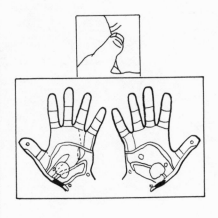

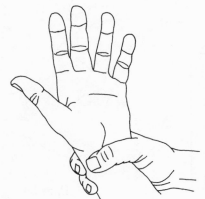

Page 82

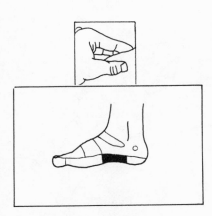

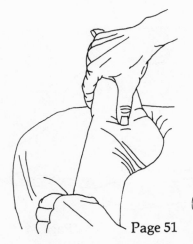

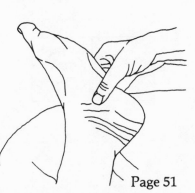

Page 51

Page 51

(continued on next page)

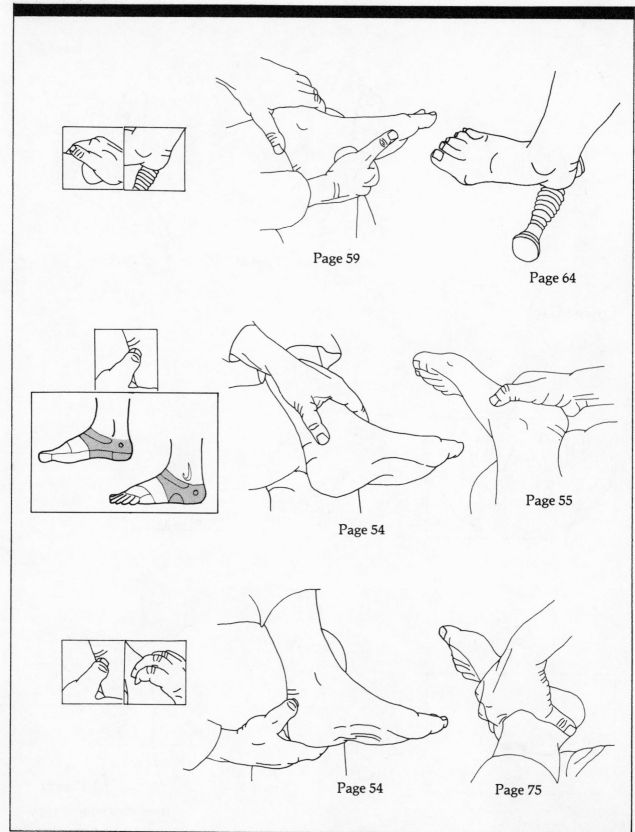

Page 59

Page 64

Page 54

Page 55

Page 54

Page 75

Tailbone

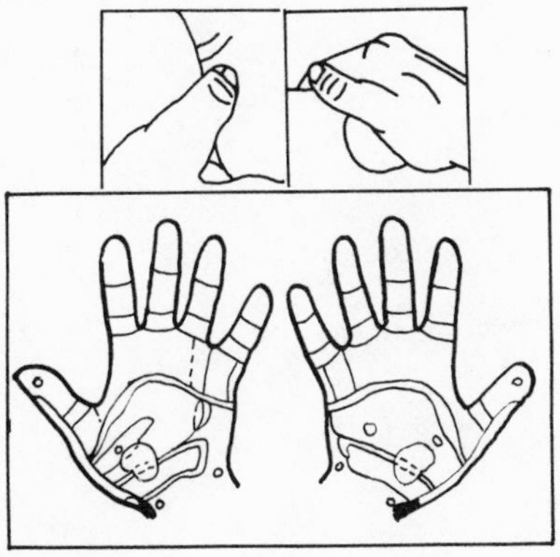

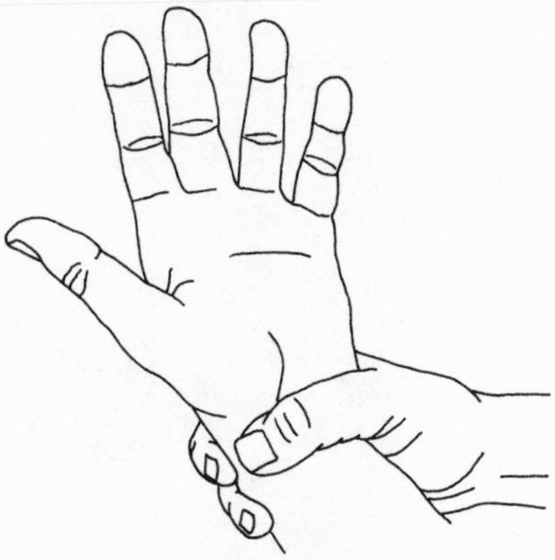

Page 82

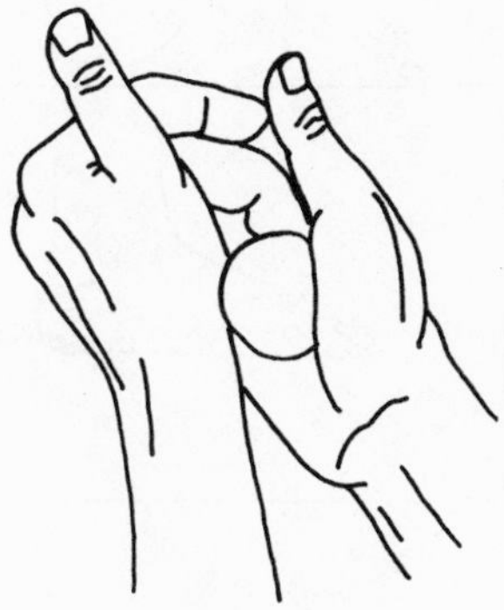

Page 89

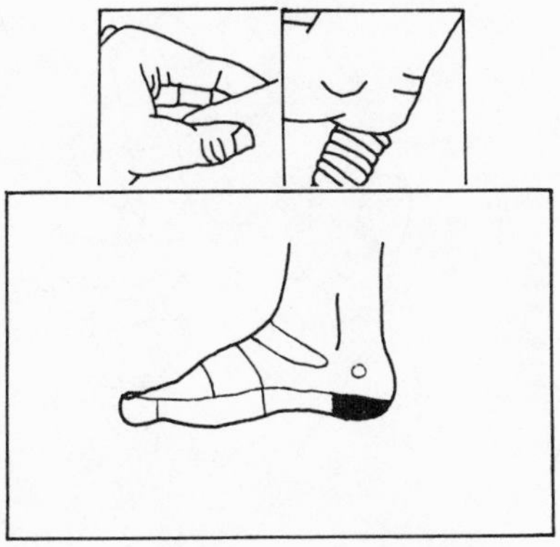

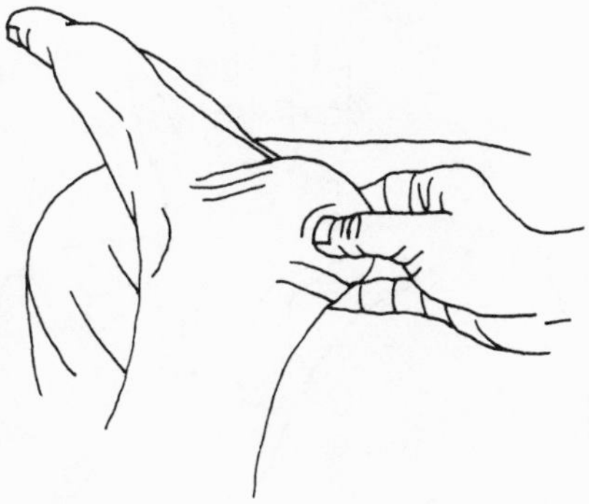

Page 51

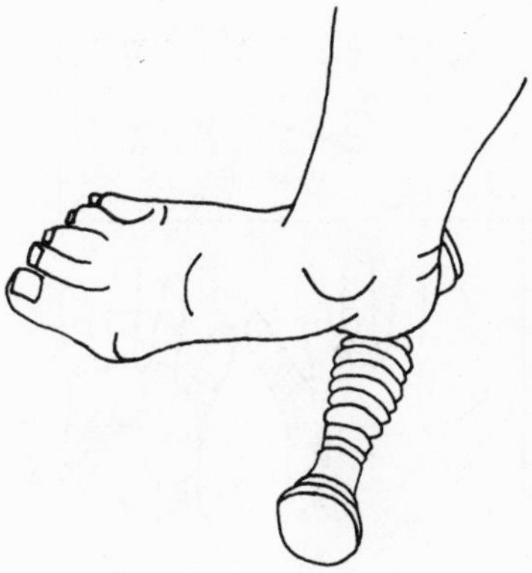

Page 64

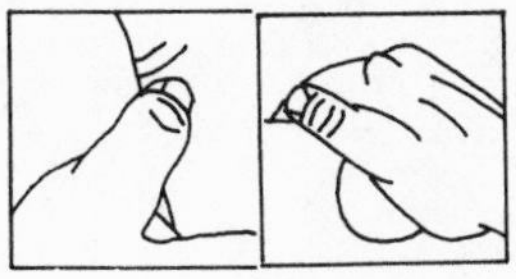

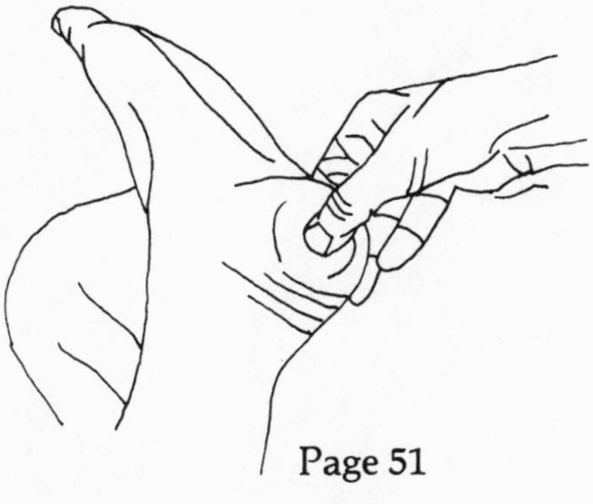

Page 51

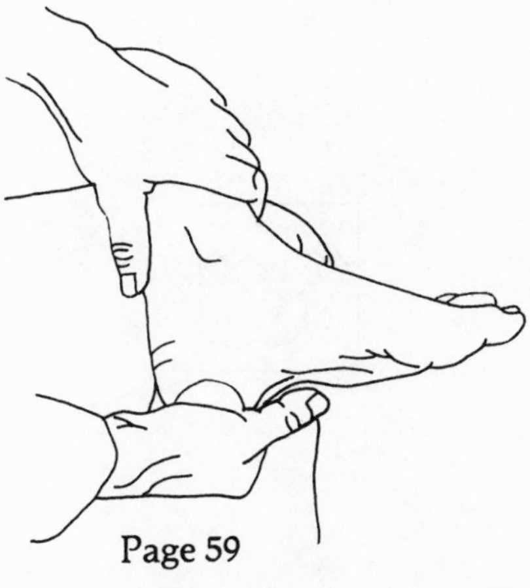

Page 59

(continued on next page)

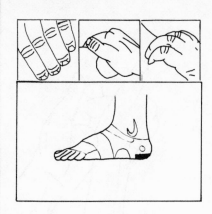

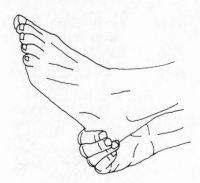

Page 52

SPLEEN

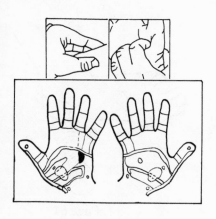

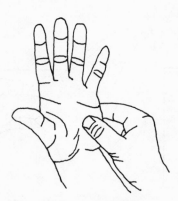

Page 71

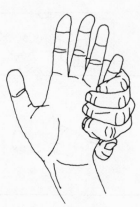

Page 75

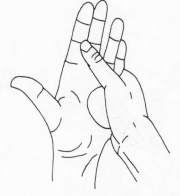

Page 89

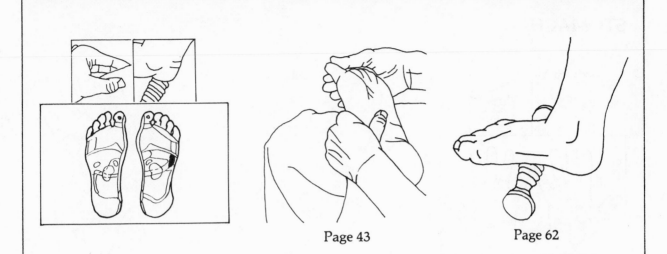

Page 43

Page 62

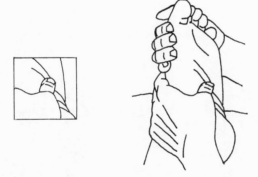

Page 46

Further Assistance:
Systems relationship: Liver

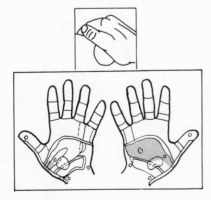

Functions include:
Involved in: infection,
blood cell quality control

STOMACH

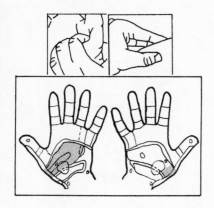

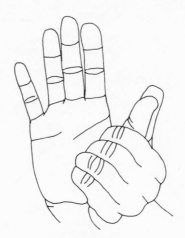

Page 74

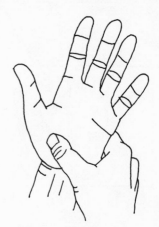

Page 71

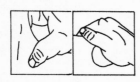

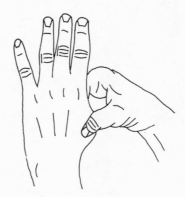

Page 78

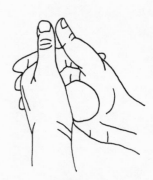

Page 89

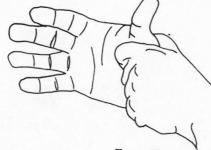

Page 76

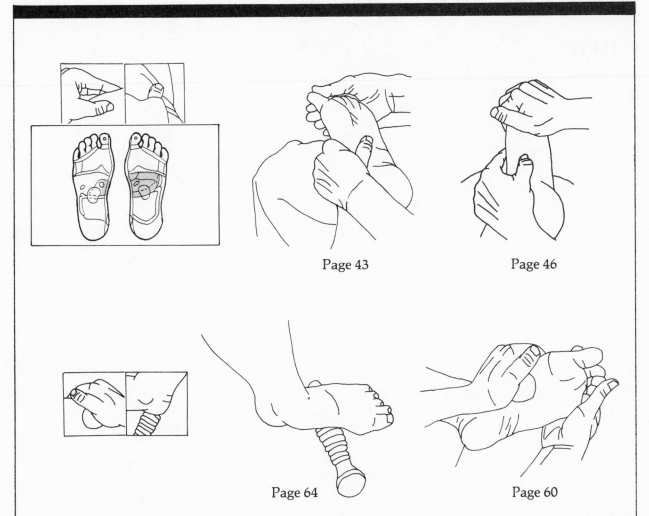

Page 43

Page 46

Page 64

Page 60

Further Assistance:
Systems relationship: Digestive system

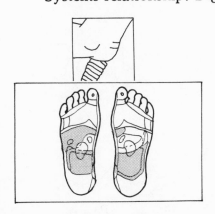

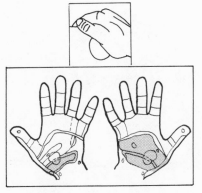

Liver, colon,
small intestine,
pancreas

TEETH

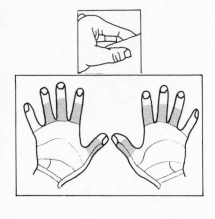

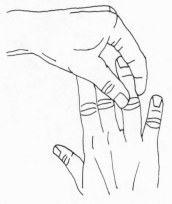

Page 83

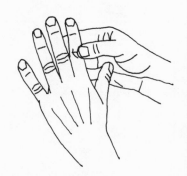

Page 79

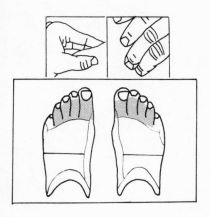

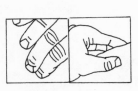

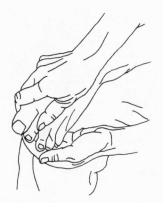

Page 47

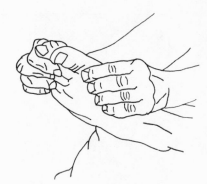

Page 47

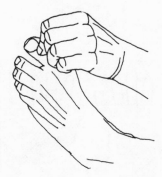

Page 47

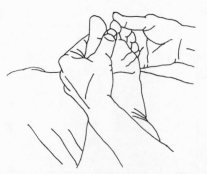

Page 42

Testicle *(See Ovary/Testicle)*

THYROID/PARATHYROID

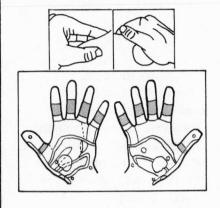

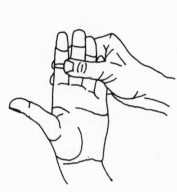

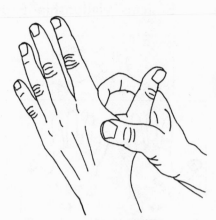

Page 70

Page 88

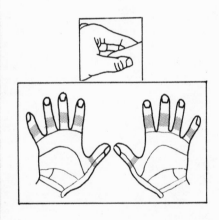

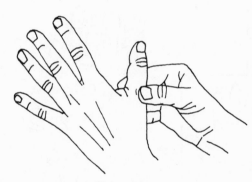

Page 79

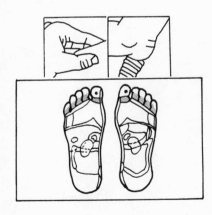

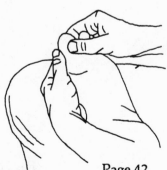

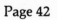

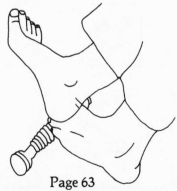

Page 42

Page 63

(continued on next page)

Further Assistance:
Systems relationship: Endocrine glands

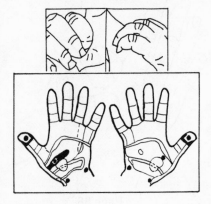

Pituitary, brain, adrenal glands, pancreas / Uterus/ prostate, ovary/testicle

Functions include:
One of the major endocrine glands.
Involved in: metabolism, dryness of skin, cholesterol, growth development, parathyroid, calcium levels, cramps

UTERUS/PROSTATE

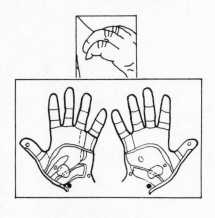

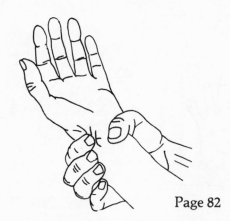

Page 82

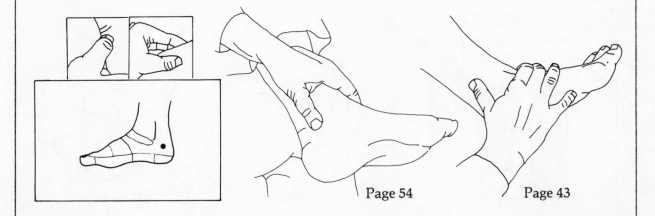

Page 54

Page 43

Further Assistance:
  Systems relationship: Endocrine glands

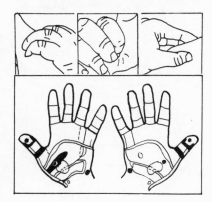

Ovary/testicle / Pituitary,
brain, adrenal glands/
pancreas / Thyroid

Further Assistance:
  Neighboring relationship: Lower back

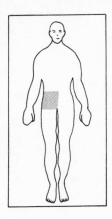 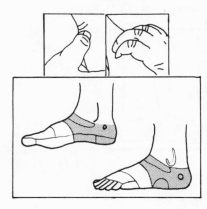

Function:
One of the major
endocrine glands.
Involved in: reproductive
capacities, maintain
sexual urge, influence
mental vigor and
physical development

WRIST

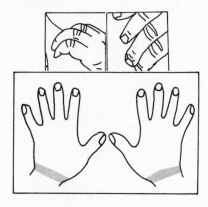

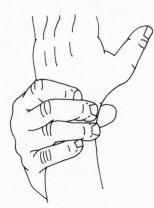

Page 82

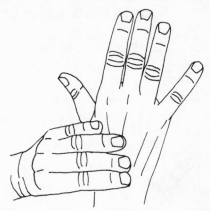

Page 80

Further Assistance:
Referral relationship: Ankle

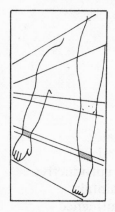

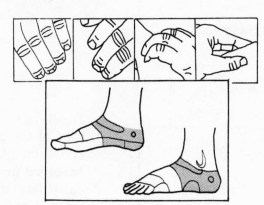

Further Assistance:
Neighboring relationship: Shoulder

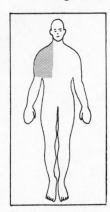

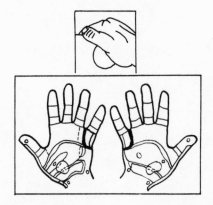

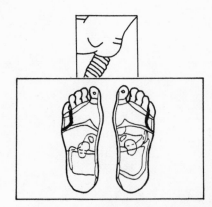

PHILOSOPHY OF SELF HELP

"All of us participate in becoming sick through a combination of mental, physical and emotional factors. You may have neglected reasonable diet, exercise or rest. You may have been very tense or anxious for a long period of time without doing enough to relax. You may have maintained unreasonable work loads or gotten so caught up in meeting everyone else's needs that you ignored your own. You may have maintained attitudes and beliefs that prevented you from having satisfying emotional experiences. In sum, you may have failed to recognize your physical and emotional limits."
Getting Well Again by O. Carl Simonton, M.D., Stephanie Matthews-Simonton, James L. Creighton, Bantam Books, New York, 1978, p.97.

Each individual has the most to say about his/her own health. Dietary considerations, exercise programs or stress reduction routines are met most effectively when directed by the individual.

Self help is a philosophy which emphasizes self-assessment as a key element in a program of wellness. Self-assessment is a major role for the body's sensory system. By using the self-perceiving mechanism, one can help adjust tension levels and/or build a more positive relationship with a body part. In other words, working on your hands and feet can give you:

- Better communication throughout the body.
- A sense that there is always a potential for change.
- A way to negate the harmful effects of stress and a method for transferring stress into a more constructive form of energy.
- A different perspective on the body, emphasizing the feet and hands as contributors to the body scheme.

Wellness can be practiced. Working on the hands and feet is a way of promoting the body's innate aptitude for feeling good. The opportunity to interact is always present.

This book is a manual of the possibilities of interaction with the hands and feet. The central theme is that *it is possible to take advantage of the way the body works and use this information for stress reduction and energy conservation.*

It is a simple, direct method of interacting with the complexities of the body. The simplicity lies in the application of sensory experience. The complexity lies in the body's interpretation of the experience.

"Something else I have learned. I have learned never to underestimate the capacity of the human mind and body to regenerate — even when the prospects seem most wretched. The life-force may be the least understood force on earth. William James said that human beings tend to live too far within self-imposed limits. It is possible that these limits will recede when we respect more fully the natural drive of the human mind and body toward perfectibility and regeneration. Protecting and cherishing that drive may well represent the finest exercise of human freedom."
Anatomy of an Illness by Norman Cousins, W.W. Norton & Co., New York, 1979, p.48.

BIBLIOGRAPHY

Cousins, Norman. *Anatomy of an Illness*, W.W. Norton and Co., New York, 1979.

Dale, Ralph Alan. *The Micro-Acupuncture Systems*, American Journal of Acupuncture, Vol. 4, No. 1, March and Vol. 4, No. 3, July-September, 1976.

Gellhorn, Ernst and Loofburrow, G.W., *Emotions and Emotional Disorders: A Neuro-Physiological Study*, Harper and Row, 1963.

Gellhorn, Ernst. *Principles of Autonomic Somatic Integration*, University of Minnesota Press, 1967.

Guyton, Arthur C., *Basic Human Physiology: Normal Function and Mechanisms of Disease*, W.B. Saunders Company, 1971.

Guyton, Arthur C., *Function of the Human Body*, W.B. Saunders Company, 1969.

Jung, Carl G., *Man and His Symbols*, Dell Publishing Co., 1968.

Miller, Jonathan. *The Body in Question*, Vintage, 1982.

Montagu, Ashley. *Touching: The Human Significance of the Skin*, Harper and Row, 1971.

Napier, John. *The Antiquity of Human Walking*, Scientific American, April 1967.

Napier, John. *The Evolution of the Hand*, Scientific American, December, 1962.

Pribram, Karl H. *Languages of the Brain: Experimental Paradoxes and Principles of Neuropsychology*, Prentice-Hall, Inc., 1971.

Selye, Hans. *Stress Without Distress*, The New American Library, Inc., 1974.

Simonton, O. Carl; Matthews-Simonton, Stephanie; Creighton, James L., *Getting Well Again*, Bantam Books, 1978.

Thompson, Richard F. *Foundation of Physiological Psychology*, Harper and Row, 1967.

INDEX

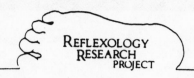

ORDER BLANK

Reflexions

        1 year subscription . . . . $12.50 _____

        Overseas subscription . . . . $18.00 _____

ART REPRODUCTIONS

_____ Set of 4 @ . . . . $4.95 ea. _____

        Postage/handling $1.25

LARGE, COLORED WALL CHART (22″ × 28″)

_____ Foot reflexology chart @ . . . . $4.95 ea. _____

_____ Hand reflexology chart @ . . . . $4.95 ea. _____

        Postage/handling $1.25

SMALL, COLORED CHART (3½″ × 6½″)

_____ Foot reflexology chart @ . . . . $2.25 ea. _____

_____ Hand reflexology chart @ . . . . $2.25 ea. _____

        Postpaid

                                         TOTAL _____

                  Check or Money Order ONLY Please

Name _____

Address _____

City _____ State_____ Zip_____

Please send a gift subscription with my compliments to:

Name _____

Address _____

City _____ State_____ Zip_____

All prices are U.S. currency and subject to change without notice.

Reflexology Research Project, P.O. Box 35820, Stn. D, Albuquerque, NM 87176